The High-Risk Neonate: Part I

Guest Editor

M. TERESE VERKLAN, PhD, CCNS, RNC

CRITICAL CARE NURSING CLINICS OF NORTH AMERICA

www.ccnursing.theclinics.com

Consulting Editor

JANET FOSTER, PhD, RN, CNS, CCRN

March 2009 • Volume 21 • Number 1

SAUNDERS an imprint of ELSEVIER, Inc.

W.B. SAUNDERS COMPANY
A Division of Elsevier Inc.

Elsevier Inc., 1600 John F. Kennedy Blvd., Suite 1800, Philadelphia, PA 19103-2899

http://www.theclinics.com

CRITICAL CARE NURSING CLINICS OF NORTH AMERICA Volume 21, Number 1
March 2009 ISSN 0899-5885, ISBN-13: 978-1-4377-0464-8, ISBN-10: 1-4377-0464-6

Editor: Katie Hartner
Developmental Editor: Donald Mumford

Critical Care Nursing Clinics of North America (ISSN 0899-5885) is published quarterly by Elsevier Inc., 360 Park Avenue South, New York, NY 10010-1710. Months of issue are March, June, September, and December. Business and Editorial Offices: 1600 John F. Kennedy Blvd., Suite 1800, Philadelphia, PA 19103-2899. Periodicals postage paid at New York, NY and additional mailing offices. Subscription prices are $130.00 per year for US individuals, $233.00 per year for US institutions, $68.00 per year for US students and residents, $167.00 per year for Canadian individuals, $292.00 per year for Canadian institutions, $191.00 per year for international individuals, $292.00 per year for international institutions and $99.00 per year for Canadian and foreign students/residents. To receive student/resident rate, orders must be accompanied by name of affiliated institution, data of term, and the signature of program/residency coordinator on institution letterhead. Orders will be billed at individual rate until proof of status is received. Foreign air speed delivery is included in all *Clinics* subscription prices. All prices are subject to change without notice. **POSTMASTER:** Send address changes to *Critical Care Nursing Clinics of North America*, Elsevier Periodicals Customer Service, 11830 Westline Industrial Drive, St. Louis, MO 63146. **Customer Service: 1-800-654-2452 (US). From outside the United States, call 1-314-453-7041. Fax: 1-314-453-5170. E-mail: JournalsCustomerService-usa@elsevier.com (for print support) and JournalsOnlineSupport-usa@elsevier.com (for online support).**

Reprints. For copies of 100 or more of articles in this publication, please contact the Commercial Reprints Department, Elsevier Inc., 360 Park Avenue South, New York, New York, 10010-1710; Tel.: (212) 633-3813, Fax: (212) 462-1935, and E-mail: reprints@elsevier.com.

Critical Care Nursing Clinics of North America is covered in *MEDLINE/PubMed (Index Medicus), International Nursing Index, Nursing Citation Index, Cumulative Index to Nursing and Allied Health Literature,* and *RNdex Top 100.*

Printed in the United States of America.

Contributors

CONSULTING EDITOR

JANET FOSTER, PhD, RN, CNS, CCRN
Assistant Professor, College of Nursing, Texas
Woman's University, Houston, Texas

GUEST EDITOR

M. TERESE VERKLAN, PhD, CCNS, RNC
Associate Professor/Neonatal Clinical Nurse
Specialist, University of Texas Health Science
Center, School of Nursing, Houston, Texas

AUTHORS

DEBBIE FRASER ASKIN, MN, RNC
Associate Professor, Faculty of Nursing;
Department of Pediatrics, Faculty of Medicine,
University of Manitoba; and Neonatal Nurse
practitioner, St. Boniface General Hospital,
Winnipeg, Manitoba, Canada

MARINA BOYKOVA, MSc, RN
Staff Nurse, Neonatal Intensive Care, Children's
Hospital #1, Saint Petersburg, Russia; and
Doctoral Student, University of Oklahoma
College of Nursing, Oklahoma City, Oklahoma

DIANNE S. CHARSHA, RN, MSN, NNP-BC
Associate Chief Nursing Officer, Cooper
University Hospital, Camden, New Jersey

SUSAN E. CHEESEMAN, RN, MSN, NNP-BC
Neonatal Nurse Practitioner, Department of
Neonatology, St. Luke's Children's Hospital,
Boise, Idaho

RUTH DAVIDGE, RN
Unit Manager, Neonatal Coordinator-Western
KZN, Greys Hospital, Pietermaritzburg
Kwazulu-Natal, South Africa

WILLIAM DIEHL-JONES, RN, PhD
Associate Professor, Faculty of Nursing;
Department of Biological Sciences, Faculty
of Science, University of Manitoba, Winnipeg,
Manitoba, Canada

CHRISTINE DOMONOSKE, PharmD
Neonatal Clinical Pharmacist, Department
of Pharmacy Services, Children's Memorial
Hermann Hospital,
Memorial Hermann Texas
Medical Center, Houston, Texas

SANDRA L. GARDNER, RN, MS, CNS, PNP
Professional Outreach Consultation, Aurora,
Colorado

MONESHA GUPTA-MALHOTRA, MBBS
Assistant Professor, Division of Cardiology,
Department of Pediatrics, University of Texas
Health Science Center, Children's Memorial
Hermann Hospital, Houston, Texas

GEORGIOS A. HARTAS, MD
Pediatric Cardiology Fellow, Division of
Cardiology, Department of Pediatrics,
University of Texas Health Science Center,
Children's Memorial Hermann Hospital,
Houston, Texas

CAROLE KENNER, DNS, RNC-NIC, FAAN
Dean/Professor, University
of Oklahoma College of Nursing;
and President, Council
of International Neonatal Nurses (COINN),
Oklahoma City, Oklahoma

CARIE E. LINDER, RNC
Certification Coordinator, Neonatal Intensive Care Unit, Integris Baptist Medical Center; and Graduate Student, Neonatal Nurse Practitioner Track, University of Oklahoma Health Science Center, College of Nursing, Oklahoma City, Oklahoma

FLORENCE MUBICHI, MS, RN
Assistant Professor, University of Oklahoma College of Nursing, Oklahoma City, Oklahoma

SHARYL L. SADOWSKI, MS, APN, NNP-BC
Neonatal Outreach Educator, Perinatal Center, Division of Obstetrics and Gynecology, University of Illinois at Chicago, Chicago, Illinois

JULIEANNE H. SCHIEFELBEIN, M App Sc, MA(Ed), Cert Hum Gen, RNM, NNP-BC, PNP-BC
Neonatal Nurse Practitioner Service (PCMC), Intermountain Health Care; Neonatal Nurse Practitioner, Primary Children's Medical Center; and Voluntary Clinical Faculty, College of Nursing, University of Utah, Salt Lake City, Utah

KAREN SEVERSON, PharmD
Pediatric Clinical Pharmacist, Department of Pharmacy Services, Children's Memorial Hermann Hospital, Memorial Hermann Texas Medical Center, Houston, Texas

NOREEN SUGRUE, PhD
Faculty Fellow, University of Oklahoma College of Nursing, Oklahoma City, Oklahoma; and Assistant Professor and Coordinator, Health and Policy Programs, Women and Gender in Global Perspectives Program, University of Illinois at Urbana-Champaign, Champaign, Illinois

EMMANOUIL TSOUNIAS, MD
Pediatric Cardiology Fellow, Division of Cardiology, Department of Pediatrics, University of Texas Health Science Center, Children's Memorial Hermann Hospital, Houston, Texas

ROBIN L. WATSON, RN, MN, CCRN
Clinical Nurse Specialist, Neonatal/Pediatrics, Harbor-UCLA Medical Center, Torrance, California

Contents

This article posits that the burden and legacy of high neonatal morbidity and mortality rates are social and economic stresses at the local, national, regional, and international levels. Furthermore, if neonatal morbidity and mortality rates are not reduced through appropriate clinical and educational means, a significant local and global consequence will be the destabilization of workforces and economies in many parts of the world. Because coordinated clinical and education efforts are required if neonatal health outcomes are to improve, and it is essential that these endeavors be led by nurses, the labor sector most likely to provide the needed care and outreach to mothers and children, a globally respected specialty nursing organization must be at the center of developing and implementing the necessary clinical and educational interventions.

Often used interchangeably, chronic lung disease (CLD) or bronchopulmonary dysplasia (BPD) develops primarily in extremely low birth weight infants weighing <1000 g who receive prolonged oxygen therapy and or positive pressure ventilation. CLD, which occurs in as many as 30 percent of infants born weighing <1000 g, contributes significantly to the morbidity and mortality seen in very low birth weight infants. Despite extensive research aimed at identifying risk factors and devising preventative therapies, many questions about the etiology and pathogenesis of BPD remain. This article reviews the embryologic development of the lung and the pathogenesis of CLD or BPD. The authors discuss some of the measures that have been used in an attempt to both prevent and treat BPD.

The subspecialty of pediatric cardiology has rapidly progressed in the past few years with more children with heart defects surviving to adulthood. With newer diagnostic tools and improved surgical techniques, many heart defects are being approached with surgery. Although, the more complicated lesions are never "completely repaired" and may require heart transplant in the long-term, there is an approach to "palliation." Most of the congenital heart malformations are detected in the perinatal period and this article gives the reader a general picture of the diagnostic approach to a multitude of heart defects.

Critical Care Nursing Clinics of North America

THE CLINICS ARE NOW AVAILABLE ONLINE!

Access your subscription at:
www.theclinics.com

Preface

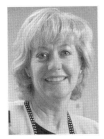

M. Terese Verklan, PhD, CCNS, RNC
Guest Editor

Advances in computers and miniaturization were key factors in taking neonatology from its pioneering phase to the sophisticated subspecialty it is today. The neonatal intensive care unit is responsible for a spectrum of ill neonates, from as young as 23 weeks' postmenstrual age (PMA) and weighing 400 g through a 41-week PMA neonate who may weigh more than 6 kg. Many intensive care units as well as special care units care for neonates who have progressed into a chronic phase of disease. Such disorders as bronchopulmonary dysplasia, intrinsic renal failure, and short-gut syndrome are not unusual sequelae and may increase the length of stay to 6 months or longer.

This is the first of two issues devoted to a review of common ailments typical of ill newborns. Dr. Kenner and colleagues begin with a discussion of global infant mortality and morbidity, with a focus on the international observations and contributions of the International Organization of Neonatal Nurses. Ms. Askin and Dr. Jones detail common respiratory problems encountered every day, along with management strategies to facilitate the neonate's recovery. Over the last few years, ventilator strategies have developed that take into consideration the neonate's own respiratory functioning. Such modalities as volume guarantee, pressure support, and synchronized intermittent mandatory ventilation have widely replaced the old standard intermittent mandatory ventilation. Although the techniques provide a kinder and gentler form of ventilation, bronchopulmonary dysplasia contributes heavily to the morbidity and mortality of extremely low birthweight survivors.

Dr. Hartas and fellow pediatric cardiologists present a well-organized approach to diagnosing cardiac disorders. Designed more for the mother-baby nurse, the assessment begins with an otherwise healthy baby, and reviews a physical examination that details what findings may be expected given a range of congenital heart defects. Often the neonatal intensive care nurse is aware of the neonate's diagnosis prior to admission. The neonate may be transferred from another facility or, if the defect is detected prenatally, the obstetrical team usually requests that the neonatal team be present at delivery to help the neonate transition successfully to extrauterine life. However, many babies with heart defects are first identified by the low-risk nursery nurse who discovers a baby in respiratory distress, who is also pale or dusky and is having difficulty feeding. A head-to-toe assessment may provide clues as to the etiology of the distress. Ms. Sadowski provides an overview of the more common congenital heart defects, along with their presentation and clinical management.

Those of you who know me, know that I have been a strong supporter of nurses attaining certification in their specialty areas. I have taught review courses for more than 10 years, as well as an item writer and member of the examination development team for both the high-risk neonate (RNC) and critical care clinical nurse specialist (CCNS) certification examinations. It gave me great pleasure to read Ms. Linder's manuscript that chronicled the path her institution took to motivate nurses to attain certification. They developed a peer-to-peer program that was essential in motivating, supporting and encouraging the nurses through the process of obtaining their specialty certification. Ms. Linder outlines how a detailed

Crit Care Nurs Clin N Am 21 (2009) ix–xi
doi:10.1016/j.ccell.2009.01.001

promotion campaign, certification packet and process was developed and implemented to keep everyone moving forward. At the completion of their first year initiative the program yielded a 38% increase in the number of certified nurses in the unit. Their overall goal is to have 59% of their eligible neonatal nurses certified, a number that places them well above the national average.

Extremely low birthweight infants weigh less than 750 g. The evidence is becoming stronger that premature preterm rupture of membranes or preterm labor is associated with an infection of the mother, such as chorioamnionitis. The resultant increased maternal proinflammatory cytokine level diffuses across the placenta and causes an increase in proinflammatory mediators in the fetus. Born so prematurely, this baby is at risk for sepsis, acute and chronic pulmonary disease, necrotizing enterocolitis, renal failure, electrolyte imbalance, hypoglycemia, and cold stress. Ms. Charsha walks the reader through the care of these tiniest patients from the delivery room through the intensive care stay.

Genetics is solving more medical mysteries as the location of genes, along with variants, are mapped. Many more tests are available to rule out metabolic and genetic disorders today than ever before. For example, phenylketonuria occurs in 1:10,000 to 15,000 live births, and is due to a defect in the activity of phenylalanine hydroxylase, the enzyme required to convert phenylalanine to tyrosine. The gene location is chromosome 12q22-q24.1. Galactosemia is the most common disorder of carbohydrate metabolism. There is a deficiency of galactose-1-phosphate-uridyltransferase such that the neonate is not able to convert galactose to glucose. Thus the neonate is not able to metabolize lactose or milk sugar, whether the milk is expressed breast milk or formulae. The gene location is chromosome 9p13. The gene has been cloned and sequenced, such that the mutations responsible for the majority of abnormalities are known. DNA sequencing and mutational analysis can be done on the parents to identify carriers and provide appropriate genetic counseling and teaching. Ms. Schiefelbein takes the reader from the science of genetics to its use at the bedside.

Few neonates escape from an intensive care or special care nursery without receiving medications, most specifically antibiotics. The increasing incidence of nosocomial infections as well as the rise of resistant microorganisms has seen a decrease in the automatic septic work-up for every admission and a concomitant decrease in antibiotic use. Despite this, the outbreaks of methicillin-resistant *Staphylococcus aureus* and vancomycin-resistant enterococci have increased. Also, more organisms are showing resistance to third-generation cephalosporins. Drs. Domonoske and Severson discuss the pharmokinetics of common medications as well as their uses for the care of the neonatal population.

Hyperbilirubinemia or jaundice is commonly diagnosed in almost every preterm neonate because of the inherent immaturity of mechanisms of conjugation of bilirubin. It was quite shocking when a number of neonates were subsequently being diagnosed with kernicterus. Kernicterus, mainly the result of overwhelming Rh disease, was thought to be a disorder of the past. Early recognition of the Rh-negative woman and effective treatment with Rhogam will prevent erythroblastosis fetalis, the main etiology for kernicterus. The Joint Commission issued a related Sentinel Event Alert in April 2001 because of the increasing number of cases being reported. It became known that the babies most affected were late-preterm infants because they were being discharged prior to the peak rise of serum total bilirubin. Since that recognition, mechanisms have been put in place to prevent the discharge of preterm neonates with increasing bilirubin levels. The next issue will contain a full discussion by Dr. Verklan in the review of the late-preterm infant. In this issue, Ms. Watson reviews the metabolism of bilirubin, the toxic effects of acute bilirubin encephalopathy if not treated, and the management of the neonate with hyperbilirubinemia.

Both preterm and term neonates have unique immunodeficiencies that predispose them to sepsis. Commonly, preterm premature rupture of membranes accompanies chorioamnionitis such that the uterine environment becomes quite hostile to the fetus, and the neonate is delivered prior to term. Clinical signs of systemic inflammation, whether suspected or proven, are common in neonatal intensive care units. Because failure to quickly treat a septic neonate increases the risk of devastating consequences, almost 50% of low–birth weight infants receive antibiotic therapy immediately after birth, even though positive blood cultures are found in only about 2% of these infants. Ms. Gardner describes the common infectious disease disorders the neonate presents with. These include group beta streptococcus and methicillin-resistant *S aureus*. She also describes the presentation, diagnostic testing, and treatment related to these disorders.

I would like to thank the contributors for sharing their expertise and experience. Many of them had just finished contributing to the text *Core Curriculum for Neonatal Intensive Care, 4th Edition* when I asked them to find the time to write yet one more manuscript. It is our hope that the reader will enjoy an up-to-date review of some of the more common and problematic areas in the realm of neonatology.

M. Terese Verklan, PhD, CCNS, RNC
Associate Professor
Neonatal Clinical Nurse Specialist
University of Texas Health Science Center
School of Nursing
6901 Bertner Avenue, Suite 565
Houston, TX 77459

E-mail address:
M.T.Verklan@uth.tmc.edu

Global Infant Mortality/ Morbidity: a Clinical Issue, a Global Organizational Approach

Carole Kenner, DNS, RNC-NIC, FAAN[a,b,]*, Noreen Sugrue, PhD[a,c],
Florence Mubichi, MS, RN[a], Marina Boykova, MSc, RN[a,d],
Ruth Davidge, RN[e]

KEYWORDS

- Neonatal global health • Workforce • Education
- Maternal-infant mortality

Evidence in developed countries supports that the more specialized training and education offered to nurses, the better the health outcomes are for all.[1] The authors contend that these improved outcomes also will accrue in developing countries if nurses receive advanced and specialized training and education. Their thoughts are premised on the knowledge that nurses in every country need specialized education and training, especially in critical care, women's health, and neonatal nursing. However, the reality is that such education and training is not provided to most nurses in developing countries. The authors propose specific policy and educational actions/steps that can be taken globally to ensure that more nurses have basic specialized training generally, specifically specialized training, and education in neonatal nursing care.

When nurses do not have sufficient specialized education and training, they are not able to meet the needs of patients. Consequences of this situation include unacceptably high rates of morbidity and mortality. When those unacceptably high rates affect women and children, especially neonates, they become a significant continuing barrier for meeting the United Nations' Millennium Development Goals (MDGs). In developing countries, the gap between the specialized education and training nurses need and what is available to them raises clinical, ethical, and policy questions requiring immediate attention. Not addressing this gap ensures that health care delivery systems will fail to meet the basic needs of patients.

The purpose of this article is to offer a model of specialized education and training for nurses in developing countries. This model may be used for any specialty area in nursing; however, in this article, the authors focus on neonatal nursing. This model provides nurses with basic specialized training and education but at the same time does

[a] University of Oklahoma College of Nursing, 1100 N. Stonewall Avenue, Oklahoma City, OK 73117, USA
[b] Council of International Neonatal Nurses (COINN), 708 Capri Place, Edmond, OK 73034, USA
[c] Women and Gender in Global Perspectives Program, University of Illinois at Urbana-Champaign, 910 South Fifth Street 320 ISB, Champaign, IL 61820, USA
[d] Neonatal Intensive Care Unit, Children's Hospital #1, 14 Avangardnaya Street, Saint Petersburg 198205, Russia
[e] Greys Hospital, PBag 9001, Pietermaritzburg Kwazulu-Natal, South Africa
* Corresponding author. Council of International Neonatal Nurses (COINN), 1100 N. Stonewall Avenue, Office 116A, Oklahoma City, OK 73117.
E-mail address: carolekenner@ouhsc.edu (C. Kenner).

Crit Care Nurs Clin N Am 21 (2009) 1–9
doi:10.1016/j.ccell.2008.09.001
0899-5885/08/$ – see front matter © 2009 Published by Elsevier Inc.

not create specialty education or training programs leading to special certification or licensing. It is important that specialized training and educational interventions for developing countries do not require special licensing or certification. First, the cost and faculty resources to offer such programs are beyond the budgetary boundaries and human resource capacity in almost all developing countries. Second, the specialized education and training should be sufficient to aid general or primary care nurses in providing fundamental specialized care to patients. This level of specialized care is likely to result in a significant and precipitous decline in morbidity and mortality rates.

The proposed model for specialized training and education in neonatal nursing care meets the clinical needs of nurses globally, will produce a decline in neonatal morbidity and mortality, and, in addition, is supported by the Council of International Neonatal Nurses (COINN). COINN is a nurse-led global organization committed to reducing neonatal, infant, and childhood morbidity and mortality through better training and education of nurses. Through case studies and exemplars, the authors present a model for delivering basic specialized training and education to neonatal nurses globally. This model can, and ought to, be used by other nursing specialty groups (eg, obstetrics, pediatrics) in order to provide nurses in developing countries with a higher level of needed training and education in specialized care.

THEORETIC FRAMEWORK

The theoretic framework underpinning this article posits that correct use and training of workers in a defined labor sector produces the best possible outcomes. The more effective a labor pool, the better the product or outcome from that labor sector. Good workers, trained and used appropriately, turn out the best outcomes. Generally, in health care, we know that the nurse is critical to good outcomes. In the United States, for example, it is recognized by the Institute of Medicine, the Magnet movement, and workforce research by Aiken and colleagues[2] that appropriately trained and educated nurses and quality nursing care are key factors for patient safety and health outcomes. The more educated the nursing workforce, the better the health outcomes[2–4] (Noreen Sugrue and Carole Kenner, unpublished data, 2008). For neonatal care and other specialty and subspecialty care, we know that nurses with some specialized training and expertise beyond a simple, or even cursory, introduction have patients with lower rates of morbidity and mortality than do the patients whose nurses have not had enhanced training and education.[2,3] For neonatal patients, that means lower rates of preventable morbidity and mortality and lower rates of long-term illnesses or disabilities, and a higher probability of living into adulthood and succeeding in school and in the workplace.

The key to achieving enhanced outcomes is better training and education of nurses and using them most effectively in clinical settings. To understand how to effect changes in the training and education of nurses within developing countries who care for neonates and infants, it is important to understand the role of nurses and the social, political, economic, and professional contexts in which these nurses work.

ROLE OF NURSES IN NONDEVELOPED COUNTRIES

Nursing shortages and underemployment/underuse of nurses are common in many developing countries. For example, a neonatal nurse was sent from Nepal to another country for specialized neonatal education but on her return to her country, her post was gone and she was assigned to work as a community health nurse. In Russia, many neonatal nurses are allowed to do only what the doctor tells them; for example, nurses may not conduct patient teaching or advocate for patients. In 2007, the Nursing Council in South Africa decided to downplay the need for neonatal trained nurses, such that nurses working on neonatal units were cast under the category of general nurses. In Kenya, nurses in Nairobi may operate as specialty nurses, yet in other parts of the country, generalized care is more likely to be encouraged and rewarded than is specialty care.

Too often, nurses are viewed as a tool to be used by doctors. Specialized nursing education and training are not thought to be necessary because it is believed that it is the doctor's expertise that is required. It is the common view that the most important influences on health outcomes are the physician's education, training, and knowledge.

NURSES AND NURSING IN RUSSIA: A CASE STUDY OF NEONATAL NURSING

Historically, Russian nurses, like nurses in most other countries, have been regarded as subservient to medicine and to physicians. In Russia, the education and training of nurses is led by medicine and physicians, and thus, nurses are taught nursing by physicians. Nurses are cast in supporting roles, whereas physicians are placed in leading roles. This traditional manner of thinking and professional socialization is challenging for nurses and physicians to overcome. It also makes it difficult for patients and ancillary health care providers not to think of nurses and nursing as secondary to physicians and medicine.

In most Russian health care facilities and on most units, including neonatal nurseries, nurses are given little autonomy and limited responsibilities. Critical and independent thinking by nurses is neither desired nor tolerated. All nursing actions are directed by medical staff. Nurses can only perform activities that are prescribed by medical doctors (eg, administer prescribed drugs or suction a baby at the time prescribed by a physician). Nurses can not formally perform health assessments because they are not taught to perform them, nor do they have the authority to conduct them. Providing information to patients is an essential part of nursing care, yet in Russia, nurses are not permitted to supply information to patients or the parents of patients. For example, in the neonatal intensive care unit (NICU), nurses may not distribute or impart information to parents. In addition, nurses are discouraged from talking with parents about the health condition of their newborns, and they are not allowed to impart health education. In developed countries, nursing documentation is essential to treat patients adequately and provide follow-up care. However, in Russia, nursing documentation consists of writing down vital signs and weight measurements, and reporting fluid balance. Nursing observations are viewed by physicians within the Russian health care system as worthless for understanding patient history, treating patients, and providing follow-up care.

In most neonatal nurseries, nurses work 24-hour shifts and are paid unduly low wages (eg, just under $500 US per month is the norm). A result of this is that nurses work second nursing jobs or non-nursing jobs in the hospital, such as housekeeper, equipment cleaner, or floor cleaner. The extra work leads to exhaustion, which eventually diminishes the nurse's effectiveness. The nurse's image as a professional health care provider who should be in partnership with the physician in caring for their patients cannot be facilitated when he/she is seen performing work in roles that require no specialized education.

Traditionally, nurses taught by doctors are trained to be physician extensions and aides. Critical thinking and independent clinical decision making are neither nurtured nor tolerated. Nurses are not seen as serious academic students and research into improving practice is nonexistent. When nurses and nursing are managed in this manner, nurses are not providing quality care and they lack foundational knowledge about neonatal nursing care. Furthermore, no administrative incentives exist for anyone to advocate for enhancing the practice of nursing. Money is lacking for nursing education and training, nursing are unwilling to take the initiative to enhance their scope of practice or to bear greater clinical responsibilities, and research and evidence-based practice data are inaccessible. In addition, one reason that nurses do not become more proactive is the lack of tolerance for the nurse advocate and educator, because the organizational culture is not supportive of independent assertive nurses or nursing practice. Health care institutions are inflexible and highly hierarchic, with nursing having no place near the apex of such a structure.

Advanced practice nursing is nonexistent in Russia. Additionally, no neonatal research or Russian language neonatal research databases exist. Nursing certification and recertification are led by commissions, which rarely contain the presence of nursing specialists on their boards. No uniform neonatal nursing practice standards or guidelines exist; moreover, no neonatal nurses associations have been established. Given this context and these working conditions, it is easy to understand how nurses working on neonatal units are undereducated and underused, and underemployed. One of these conditions by itself may lead to low morale, high turnover, and unacceptably high morbidity and mortality rates, and, placed in combination, the effects are devastating to the profession's advancement. Not only do the conditions obstruct the development of neonatal nursing in Russia, they hinder the possibility that the highest quality nursing care is ever going to be available to patients and create obstacles/impasses to evidence-based nursing practice in Russia.

One way to combat the undereducation and underemployment of nurses is international connections and collaborations, which are important if delivery of continuing education and training is to occur. The strategy is also essential as a means of creating professional networks and increasing professional motivation, self-awareness, assertiveness, confidence, and empowerment. Nursing in Russia, like in most developing countries, requires a pool of motivated nurses if the practice of nursing is to evolve. These nurses must be able to develop strategies to enhance collaboration and professional networking.

In addition, in order for specialty nursing to take hold and lead to practice improvement, a forum must exist for nurses to learn, develop a vision for the future, and advocate for themselves and their patients. Nurses working in specialty areas must create a professional community that advocates for the educational and professional advancement of nurses. Nurses in developing countries require international collaboration with nurses and nursing organizations that face similar struggles and those that can provide support and guidance. In short, specialty nurses in developing countries need access to nurses and nursing organizations in other developing countries and to those in developed nations. For neonatal nurses, international collaboration through organizations such as COINN provides access to nurses working and facing challenges in developing countries and to those working and facing challenges in developed countries. Such an international organization provides access to ideas, education modules, research, and the potential for collaborative engagement. The organization, and others like it, provides nurses with the opportunity to improve their own knowledge and skill base and the practice of nursing within their own countries.

UNITED STATES–RUSSIA COLLABORATION

One long-term international project has brought a distinctive improvement in neonatal care. The collaboration involved the NICU of Children's Hospital #1 of Saint Petersburg, Russia (CH#1), three other NICUs in Saint Petersburg, and the Children's Hospital of Oakland (CHO) in Oakland, California. This collaboration focused on the professional development of nurses. In 1987, prior to the collaboration, the mortality rate of newborns in the NICU stood at 33%, and the mortality rates for those weighing less than 2000 grams was 80%.[5]

The Russian NICU Program started in 1990 when the first visit from the American team took place. At that time, CH#1 had 12 NICU beds. Small budgets and the absence of sophisticated high-tech devices meant that the unit was scarcely equipped. In 1990, the unit's mortality rate was about 25% and it had an annual census of approximately 350. At that time, the Russian nurses were given 2 months of in-service, or on-the-job, training in neonatal intensive care nursing, which followed basic nursing training provided by physicians at the hospital. The basics of normal or well baby care are taught at nursing schools in Russia but in 1990, and still today, no neonatal specialty training for nurses exists. Yet for more than 15 years, neonatal care and outcomes have improved in Russia; this improvement is due to the effective international collaboration between CH#1 and CHO.

As patient management and care improved, the number of admissions at the Russian NICU increased almost fourfold, whereas the length of hospital stay and morbidity decreased significantly.[5] The mortality rate of neonates weighing less than 2000 grams decreased to 8.8% in 2004 and mortality rates of all neonates in the NICU decreased to 5.7% in 2005.[5] The positive results achieved at the largest NICU in the city also influenced neonatal care throughout the city of Saint Petersburg. Because of the trickle-down effect of the knowledge, and the decrease in early neonatal mortality, overall infant mortality has significantly declined in Saint Petersburg since CH#1 and CHO established their international collaboration. Today, Saint Petersburg has an infant mortality rate of 7.1 per 1000 live births, the lowest infant mortality rate in the Russian Federation.[6]

These achievements were accomplished, quite simply, through respectful, continuous collaborative work between health care providers in a developed nation and those in a less developed or developing country. In the case of the United States–Russia collaboration, the American team, consisting of nurses and doctors and other health care specialists (about 10 to 15 people) visited Saint Petersburg for 2 weeks of intensive training, education, and clinical work. Although the collaboration was with CH#1, health care providers from any facility in Saint Petersburg were permitted to participate with, and learn from, the members of the American team. Early in the collaboration, visits by the American team occurred twice a year, and this gradually decreased to once a year. During the project, many different medical specialists visited NICUs in Russia (eg, neonatologists, perinatologists, pediatric surgeons, and obstetricians). Visiting perinatal and neonatal nurses included clinical nurse specialists, nurse managers, those with expertise in infection control, and transport nurses. The visiting American team also included respiratory therapists and biomedical engineers.

Every day that the American team was present, American and Russian physicians and nurses participated in clinical rounds. Physicians and nurses worked together to learn how to best provide the necessary neonatal care. In addition, on a daily basis, the American team members conducted educational activities, including seminars and lectures on clinical issues, patient management, and new technologies in the field of neonatal care. These activities were free and easily accessible, not trivial concerns for nurses whose salaries are low and for whom continuing education resources are nonexistent. In practice and theory, American nurses and physicians taught their Russian counterparts how to work as a collaborative interdisciplinary team, and introduced new clinical skills such as percutaneous silastic intravenous line insertion, aspects of caring for extremely low birth weight babies, and new wound care approaches.

Incorporating this knowledge into routine NICU care contributed to the declining neonatal and infant morbidity and mortality rates that has occurred in Saint Petersburg over the last 15 to 18 years.

In addition to training and education, the American team provided essential technical support. At the beginning of the project, the American team brought basic humanitarian aid to the Russian NICU at CH#1, which included incubators, ventilators, pulse oximeters, basic supplies, and other equipment. The supplies were collected from a number of hospitals in the United States specifically for the Russian NICUs. At that time, the equipment was not widely available to Russian NICUs, and even if it were, the costs would have been prohibitive. With time, as the technical base in Russia improved, the American team brought other the valuable pieces of equipment, such as neonatal and perinatal educational materials, books, protocols, and standards of care used in the hospitals in the United States. The fact that the materials were given free to Russian participants was of major importance to Russian nurses because their salaries were too low to enable them to purchase these materials on their own.

Another aspect was important in the success of the collaborative effort in diminishing neonatal mortality in Russia. During the years of the project, not only did the American team visit Russia, but Russian doctors and nurses also visited hospitals in the United States. These visits were sponsored by American colleagues. The Russian team included neonatal nurses and physicians from different children's hospitals and maternity houses in Saint Petersburg. During the period from 1991 to 2002, approximately 20 Russian health care providers visited the NICU of CHO.

Another important note is that the project received support from both the Russians and the Americans. It was supported by the Saint Petersburg Department of Health and, in the United States, by the East Bay Neonatology Foundation in California. Leaders from the Saint Petersburg Department of Health and the government of Saint Petersburg realized the importance of education and training of health care personnel, and provided financial and political support for this project. This project began during "perestroika," when the climate in the country promoted change and development, a sense of optimism existed, people were encouraged to work together despite economic and financial difficulties, and implementing new ideas and technologies was rewarded. This context was a necessary, but not sufficient, condition for a successful collaboration.

Between 1993 and 1994, a reconstruction took place at the NICU at Children's Hospital #1, which also influenced the results from the Russian NICU unit. The unit was rebuilt, the bed capacity increased from 12 to 30 beds (24 beds with ventilators), the number of nursing personnel increased from 24 to 144, and the technical conditions of the unit improved (eg, centralized vacuum and oxygen supply, several sinks, floor, lighting). The unit's reconstruction was sponsored by American colleagues ($25,000 US) and the Saint Petersburg Department of Health ($15,000 US). In 1998, a special federal program, "Provision of guaranteed care for newborns of Saint Petersburg," provided new equipment to the NICUs of the city. Eight million American dollars were spent for new monitors, ventilators, infusion pumps, and incubators, all of which helped improve care for newborns in the city[7] (A. D'Harlingue and C. Lund, personal communication, 2008). Now the NICU at Children's Hospital #1 had the necessary technical components for providing up-to-date neonatal care.

What were the reasons for success during the collaboration project with the American team? The facts and numbers do not tell the entire story of what happened during the last 15 to 18 years of the project. The project was unusual in terms of its longevity because, typically, most international projects usually last for only a few years. From the personal point of view of one of the authors (M. Boykova), a central ingredient for the project's success was learning as one practiced at the bedside. Learning at the bedside allowed for real patient care problems to be discussed and resolved. The scenario also taught nurses how to make clinical decisions, act in the patient's best interest, and work within an interdisciplinary team. Although different conferences in Russia and abroad provided a valuable role in the improvement of care, the close and practical communication next to the patient played a significant part. The importance of the presence of nurse collaborators on the unit cannot be overstated. Interdisciplinary clinical rounds, discussions, and collaboration, and acquiring skills and knowledge about the complexities of neonatal care are factors that all led to the success of the project.

It was important that practical, everyday clinical issues were combined with educational and research seminars and lectures given by American nurses and doctors. It linked theory, research, and practice. If the project was only to demonstrate American practices or to showcase humanitarian aid in the form of new equipment or medications, the project would not have achieved the success it did; far too many examples of such international projects exist and the results from them are less than stellar. The exchange of practical knowledge and experience, and providing educational opportunities, were two main factors that influenced the success of this project.

The third, and perhaps even most important, factor for success was that the interdisciplinary team approach was used. Too often, international collaborations are disciplinary or practice specific and do not incorporate an interdisciplinary model of training and education that includes physicians and nurses together. As anyone who has clinical experience knows, good patient outcomes require interdisciplinary cooperation and coordination. For almost all hospital situations, it is the bedside nurse who has the most in-depth knowledge of the patient and his/her condition. Nurses are with the patients more than any other health care provider. Positive interdisciplinary work produced some changes in the Russian NICU because more cooperation existed and the nurses' attitudes towards physicians appeared to be less subservient. Despite those positive experiences, the organizational culture and professional socialization are slow to change and, unfortunately, the level of physician–nurse cooperation and respect in Russian NICUs remains significantly lower than was anticipated, given this project.

The final factor in the success of the program was consistency. Consistency and continuity of visits by the same American team members interacting with the same Russian team members positively influenced the development of understanding and a relationship between two groups. Because this continuity avoided repetition of some of the concepts, terms, and issues, it resulted in efficient and effective short-term teaching modules.

WHY PROVIDING NURSES WITH ENHANCED TRAINING AND EDUCATION IN NEONATAL CARE IS REQUIRED IN DEVELOPING COUNTRIES

The Russian example supports the notion of professional education being tied to improved neonatal outcomes. Most neonatal and infant mortality is due to preventable causes such as infection, diarrhea, and nutrition. Another issue is the fact that pregnant women experience poor weight gain and continue to do hard manual labor, which contribute to the birth of premature and low–birth-weight infants.[8] Distances to health care facilities are great, often taking 3 to 4 hours by car, if one is available, on hard, treacherous roads.

In Kenya, the health problems focus on HIV, malaria, tuberculosis, malnutrition, and the lack of clean water. Tribal conflicts this past year have also resulted in less travel by some women. The spread of mosquito netting, along with education about the connection between the mosquito bite and the transmission of malaria, are beginning to have an impact. Increasing education for women is making a difference because women are the health care decision makers for the family. Another aspect of life that has changed is the emphasis on the use of nonnutritive sucking to stimulate growth, better nutrition, and the sanitation of water. The last two factors are being addressed by the World Health Organization's (WHO) Partnership in Safe Motherhood and Newborn Health, which addresses the MDGs.

The United Nations Children's Fund (UNICEF), along with other organizations such as COINN, is working to address the issues identified in the Neonatal Survival series published by *Lancet* in 2005, which challenged the world to combat the preventable causes of neonatal morbidity and mortality.[9] It was reported that about 2 million babies die within the first 24 hours of life and a total of 4 million die within the neonatal period, thus accounting for almost 40% of all childhood deaths globally.[9] Most of the interventions that are required to reduce morbidity and mortality do not, as indicated by the Russian and Kenyan examples, require high technology. They require education and training in simple things, such as how to teach families about proper nutrition, the importance of clean water, hand washing, thermoregulation or warming of an infant, and the impact of the environment, particularly on an immature immune system as found in the premature, or even the term, neonate. Use of techniques such as nonnutritive sucking, swaddling, and kangaroo care are all nontechnical interventions that may save lives.

Teaching neonatal resuscitation and stabilization techniques is good but must be done within the context of available equipment and medications. The American Academy of Pediatrics and the American Heart Association have begun instructing health care providers throughout the world on how to use the Neonatal Resuscitation Programs and STABLE. Some cultures are concerned about implementing them fully in clinical use because they do not have all the equipment or medications recommended in the programs. The March of Dimes has a globalization arm that is working with UNICEF and others to improve maternal child outcomes. The Gates Foundation has supported projects in Africa aimed at decreasing HIV. Most of these interventions require little technology but rely on sweat equity for training of the trainer to engage the community for long-term sustainability. For example, in Kenya, when mosquito netting was delivered by an overseas organization with no training given on how to use it, the netting had no effect. Once local health professionals became involved in teaching the population about malaria and infection control and the relationship of the disease to mosquito netting use, the proper use increased and infections decreased. The WHO and the International Council of Midwives have worked towards training skilled birth attendants. Although these are lay helpers, they are successful in the bush in Africa or in rural villages in Asia where, as a rule, women deliver in the home rather than the hospital. For example, skilled birth attendants are present at 54% of all the births in Malawi.[10]

The health of women and children, particularly infants, reflects on a nation's commitment to the health and welfare of all its citizens in that how a nation treats its most vulnerable and least powerful reflects its commitment to the care of its people. The moral, social, familial, economic, and community prices paid for premature morbidity and mortality among neonates is too high; nations cannot afford to "lose" these people. UNICEF,[11] when working with water sanitization projects, found that for every 10% increase in female literacy, a country's economic growth was increased by 0.3%. Educated women are more likely to raise healthier families, and the rates of AIDS, general infections, and malnutrition are likely to decrease. Lowering infant mortality also enhances a family's ability to invest in health and education, and vice versa.[11] The moral, social, family, economic, and community factors highlight the role of training and education of nurses in order to meet the MDGs. Without enhanced training and education of nurses, MDGs 4 and 5 (reduction of maternal and childhood mortality rates) will not be met. If the morbidity and mortality of women and children are not reduced, precious little chance exists that the other MDGs can subsequently be met. Expanded training and education of nurses in neonatal care is a necessary condition for meeting the MDGs.

HOW TO PROVIDE THE ENHANCED TRAINING AND EDUCATION: COUNCIL OF INTERNATIONAL NEONATAL NURSES AS THE EXEMPLAR

COINN was formed over the last decade to improve maternal and infant outcomes and represents national organizations that support neonatal nursing care. It began with the union of the United Kingdom, Australian, New Zealand, and United States neonatal nursing associations. It now has grown to include many other organizational members, including groups in Canada, South Africa, and India, that it helped start. Fifty countries are represented through its regional networks. COINN's mission is to foster excellence in neonatal nursing, promote the development of neonatal nursing as a recognized global specialty, create high standards for neonatal care, enhance the quality of care for patients and families, decrease health disparities, and improve outcomes. The vision is to promote global unity in neonatal nursing. The work is done through building capacity at the country level.

In its work with the WHO and the International Council of Nurses, where it is an affiliate member, COINN has been invited to the policy table to work with world leaders to promote neonatal nursing practice and education standards. In 2007, COINN, with support from UNICEF and the Minister of Women and Children's Health, helped charter the India Association of Neonatal Nurses. The Neonatology Forum, a physician group, also supported this move because they felt that the only way to impact neonatal outcomes was to improve the status and education of Indian nurses. COINN is also working with the neonatal association in South Africa to regain recognition for neonatal nursing as a specialty. The Neonatal Nursing Association of South Africa will create standards and guidelines for neonatal nursing education and care.

Since the early 1970s, neonatal nursing in the United States, and subsequently in Australia, Canada, and New Zealand, has been recognized as a specialty with either training in the neonatal unit or a master of science in nursing specialized programs. These countries recognize that caring for children requires different skills than caring for adults. Another outcome of this professional association movement has been to recruit and retain more nurses in neonatal care. All nurses are not equally prepared after basic education to provide specialized care to neonates. Specialty training is required, either on the job or in a professional educational program, with credentials provided by experts in the field.

Neonatal care should be provided as a first-line defense in health care because this is more cost effective than emergency, critical, or long-term care. For instance, the direct health care cost of an intensive care treatment is cheaper than long-term treatment cost because if treatment is delayed, these babies often require more sophisticated treatment and care, which places additional financial burden on a country. So, given this example, where does this leave us in terms of neonatal care?

SUGGESTED POLICIES

The Russian case is illustrative of what is found in too many countries, especially those with a developing economy. As the Russian example shows, the education and training of nurses, changing the culture of a physician-dominated health care system, addressing nursing shortages, and the overall economic barriers to providing care will not disappear or be "fixed" immediately. Therefore, any policy responses must be tailored to take into account these conditions/contexts. With that in mind, the following policy suggestions seem workable and are likely to lead to improved outcomes; however, these are not the ideal solutions or the end-stage ones, and should be seen as a starting point.

  Globally, create incentives for health care systems in developing countries to encourage, seek out, and support intensive nursing specialty short courses. These courses should include nurses, physicians, and other health care providers as equal participants. The purpose of the courses is to impart technical and clinical knowledge but also to teach interdisciplinary team work to all health care providers.

  Developed countries, as part of their bilateral aid programs/packages, should support specialty nursing groups and organizations in developing short courses related to nursing care that can be administered face to face and on video. This condition is necessary because teams from developed countries cannot always be present in developing nations and yet the nurses in those countries may need more information and training than is available to them during the short intensive visits by teams from developed nations.

  Any global or bilateral aid package should include enhanced short-term exchange programs whereby nurses from less developed and developing countries are sent to developed countries for short, intensive, specialized nursing training and education in neonatal, women's health, and critical care. At the same time, nurses from developed nations would be sent to less developed and developing nations to teach intensive, short courses in specialized nursing care. This policy will require creativity and flexibility in practice boundaries, at least temporarily. In order for the exchange to work, licensing exceptions will needed on the part of all participating countries or the clinical component of these short-term intensive courses cannot be implemented. These short courses require that nurses have a clinical component to the education and training.

  Developed, less developed, and developing nations all need to commit to providing the technologic infrastructure to nurses in the less developed and developing nations. The infrastructure should also include regular access to Wi-Fi. This infrastructure commitment is necessary if nurses, on a continuing basis, are to have access to data, research, experts, and online education modules.

  Developed countries should support the work of one international nursing organization devoted to each of the following specialty areas: neonatal care, women's health, and critical care; the purpose of the support is to ensure the development, coordination, and implementation of collaborative short-term intensive training and education for nurses. This support would further ensure that the educational efforts would be continuous and that the development of collaborating partnerships between less developed and developing nations on one hand and developed nations on the other would be supported technically, politically, professionally, and perhaps economically.

  International nursing organizations that focus on one nursing specialty or subspecialty (eg, neonatal care, critical care, women's health) must develop short-term courses and case studies that detail best clinical practices in order to provide nurses in less developed and developing nations with the specialized education and training that will allow them to better meet the needs of their patients. The nurses in need of this training and education are not able to spend the requisite time in graduate school to acquire a specialized certificate or diploma; moreover, the countries where most of these nurses live do not have the economic, education, or human capital needed to provide nurses with specialty training. These short courses are the most viable training and education options for nurses in less developed and developing nations who need specialty training.

Taken together, these policy recommendations are designed to enhance the knowledge and clinical specialty skills of nurses in developing and less developed nations; besides the normative and moral imperative of noblesse oblige, developed nations have a vested interest in terms of economic, political, and social stability, to ensure that the health of those living in poorer nations improves.

None of the proposed policies, in and of themselves or as a package, are cost prohibitive and, taken together, they are likely to improve the overall health of patients and the clinical skills of many providers. In short, implementing these policies is likely to result in a decrease in morbidity and mortality. The policy recommendations do not alter the educational design or administrative structure of health care delivery in any country; rather, they provide a way to deliver to nurses the necessary specialized education and training they need to better meet the needs of their patients.

SUMMARY

Neonatal nurses cannot do it all. The enhanced training and education suggested for them is one piece of a complex puzzle that needs to be put together in order to improve the health of people globally. Such enhanced training and education must be carried out in several nursing specialty and subspecialty areas. The contribution of this article is in recognizing and arguing for some level of specialized training and education for nurses, but acknowledging that it must be more of a continuing education/continuing medical education model or curriculum, rather than formal graduate education. In developing and less developed countries, the workforce capacity, educational infrastructure, labor pool, and health care infrastructure do not warrant an advanced training and education model for nurses other than one that is similar to that proposed in this article. If such a model were implemented, it would increase the likelihood that the MDGs would be met, the health and welfare of all people would improve, and preventable morbidity and mortality would decrease. However, these dramatic changes will occur only when all nurses, not just neonatal nurses, in developing countries have access to more and continuous training and education in specialty and subspecialty areas of care.

The other consideration underscored in this article is the importance of correctly identifying the roles and responsibilities of nurses. This condition is necessary if health outcomes and clinical resources are to be maximized. The situation in developing and less developed countries tends to highlight the need to reassess the nurses' roles and responsibilities. The reassessment is necessary if we truly are to alter morbidity and mortality rates and use health care resources in the most effective and efficient manner. At the same time, health care and political leaders in developed and developing countries need to acknowledge that maximizing the training and education of nurses, especially in specialty and subspecialty areas, while also clarifying their roles and responsibilities, ensuring the development of independent and critical thinking skills, and guaranteeing autonomous working conditions are necessary conditions for the optimal use of health care resources, including health care labor, in order to improve health outcomes.

REFERENCES

1. United Nations. UN millennium development goals, 2008. Available at: http://www.un.org/millenniumgoals/index.html#. Accessed June 22, 2008.
2. Aiken LH, Clarke SP, Sloane DM, et al. Effects of hospital care environment on patient mortality and nurse outcomes. J Nurs Adm 2008;38(5):223–9.
3. Institute of Medicine (IOM). Keeping patients safe: transforming the work environment of nurses. Washington, DC: National Academies Press; 2004.
4. Dunton N, Gajewski B, Klaus S, et al. The relationship of nursing workforce characteristics to patient outcomes. OJIN 2007;12(3). Available at: http://www.nursingworld.org/MainMenuCategories/ANAMarketplace/ANAPeriodicals/OJIN/TableofContents/Volume122007/No3Sept07/NursingWorkforceCharacteristics.aspx#IOM04. Accessed June 22, 2008.
5. Lubimenko VA. Annual report, NICU, Children's Hospital #1 2005. Saint Petersburg, Russia.
6. Shabalov NP. Neonatology. 4th edition. Moscow: MED press-inform; 2006.
7. Khodireva GA, Kokareva TG, Kuznetsova EU. Present state and perspectives for development of hospital care for children of Saint Petersburg. Detskaya bolnitsa 2002;3(9):7–9.
8. Mubichi F, Kenner C. International connections: Kenyan neonatal morbidity and mortality: genetics or not? Newborn Infant Nurs Rev 2008;8(1):e25–6.
9. Lawn JE, Cousens S, Zupan J, for the Lancet Neonatal Survival Steering Team. Neonatal survival 1: 4 million neonatal deaths: when? Where? Why? Lancet 2005;365(9462):891–900.
10. UNICEF. Malawi. Available at: http://www.unicef.org/infobycountry/malawi_statistics.html. Accessed June 22, 2008.
11. UNICEF. Why sanitation is important for children. Available at: http://www.unwater.org/worldwaterday/docs/kids-sanitation.pdf. Accessed June 22, 2008.

Pathogenesis and Prevention of Chronic Lung Disease in the Neonate

Debbie Fraser Askin, MN, RNC[a,b,d,]*, William Diehl-Jones, RN, PhD[a,c]

KEYWORDS

- Bronchopulmonary dysplasia • Chronic lung disease
- Neonate • Premature

Increased survival rates in infants born between 24 and 26 weeks gestation has resulted in larger numbers of neonates who require respiratory support at birth. Despite the use of antenatal steroids, exogenous surfactant, and a variety of modes of ventilation, a number of these neonates develop complications of prematurity, including the development of chronic lung disease (CLD). Often used interchangeably, CLD or bronchopulmonary dysplasia (BPD) develops primarily in extremely low birth weight infants (ELBW) weighing <1000 g who receive prolonged oxygen therapy and or positive pressure ventilation.[1] CLD, which occurs in as many as 30 percent of infants born weighing <1000 g, contributes significantly to the morbidity and mortality seen in very low birth weight infants.[2]

Despite extensive research aimed at identifying risk factors and devising preventative therapies, many questions about the etiology and pathogenesis of BPD remain. It is known that acute lung injury, resulting from a multitude of factors including the pressure, volume and oxygen associated with mechanical ventilation, initiates a cascade of inflammation, arrested lung development, and abnormal repair processes that ultimately damage the still-immature alveoli and result in prolonged oxygen dependency. This article reviews the embryologic development of the lung and the pathogenesis of CLD or BPD. The authors discuss some of the measures that have been used in an attempt to both prevent and treat BPD.

DEFINING BPD

BPD was first described by Northway and colleagues[3] in 1967. At that time, neonates with severe respiratory distress syndrome (RDS) were treated with conventional mechanical ventilation using high peak inspiratory pressures and high levels of inspired oxygen. These infants remained oxygen dependent beyond the expected resolution of their RDS, had acute episodes of bronchospasm, and demonstrated classic radiographic changes, including the presence of areas of atelectasis and cystic hyperinflation.[3] Northway and colleagues[3] developed a set of criteria for both defining and staging the severity of BPD. In this staging system, Stage I and II BPD occurred in the first ten days of life with the findings indistinguishable from RDS. Stage III marked the transition to chronic disease and Stage IV occurred in infants who, at one month of age continued to require oxygen or ventilatory support and who associated radiographic abnormalities.

Building on the work of Northway, Bancalari and colleagues[4] suggested additional clinical criteria to support a diagnosis of BPD: ventilation for a minimum of three days in the first week of life; and, at 28 days of life, the need for supplemental oxygen to maintain oxygen levels of at least 50 mm Hg, clinical signs of respiratory distress (tachypnea, retractions, adventitious breath sounds) and an abnormal chest radiograph.

[a] Faculty of Nursing, University of Manitoba, Winnipeg, Manitoba, Canada
[b] Department of Pediatrics, Faculty of Medicine, University of Manitoba, Winnipeg, Manitoba, Canada
[c] Department of Biological Sciences, Faculty of Science, University of Manitoba, Winnipeg, Manitoba, Canada
[d] St. Boniface General Hospital, Winnipeg, Manitoba, Canada
* Corresponding author.
E-mail address: debbie_fraser@umanitoba.ca (D.F. Askin).

Crit Care Nurs Clin N Am 21 (2009) 11–25
doi:10.1016/j.ccell.2008.09.006
0899-5885/08/$ – see front matter © 2009 Elsevier Inc. All rights reserved.

More recently, the introduction of antenatal steroids, exogenous surfactant therapy, synchronized modes of ventilation, and aggressive nutritional support have changed the course of the ELBW infant and of BPD. The classic or "old BPD" seen in both preterm and term infants, had been replaced by a "new BPD" seen almost exclusively in ELBW neonates. This new BPD is less severe and, in many cases, presents in infants who had mild lung disease and required little or no supplemental oxygen at birth.[5] The newer type of CLD highlights the need to re-examine the definition of BPD. Some studies done in the 1980s and 1990s used the need for oxygen at 28 days to define BPD;[6,7] however, this definition would include infants who may have an acute illness at that time and may exclude neonates who subsequently require supplemental oxygen.[5] Other criteria used to define BPD include the need for supplemental oxygen at 36 weeks postconceptual age[8] or the presence of chronic respiratory symptoms requiring treatment in the first year or two of life.[9,10]

In 2000, the National Institutes of Health (NIH) held a consensus conference for the purpose of identifying a common definition of BPD. The result was a list of diagnostic criteria that is based on the need for supplemental oxygen for a minimum of 28 days. The amount of oxygen needed is used to determine the severity of disease (**Table 1**).[11] Although this definition has become widely accepted, it has not yet been prospectively evaluated.[12]

INCIDENCE

Variable definitions and inclusion criteria make it difficult to determine the incidence of BPD. Even in multisite studies using a common definition, the incidence of BPD varies widely among sites.[12,13] Walsh and colleagues[14] identified an incidence of 35% in their study of 1598 low birth weight (LBW) infants (<1250 g), while Sahni and group[15] found that only 7.4% of infants in their study needed oxygen at 36 weeks postconceptual age.

When the NIH definition of BPD was applied in a retrospective review of 4866 ELBW infants done by Ehrenkranz and colleagues,[16] they found that 77 percent of the neonates met the NIH criteria for BPD with 16 percent having severe disease and 30% moderate BPD.

PATHOGENESIS

BPD has been associated with lung inflammation and fibrosis, and BPD was presumed to primarily reflect barotraumas secondary to mechanical ventilation. The lungs of infants who have BPD presented with signs of infection, inflammation, and parenchymal fibrosis; otherwise, areas devoid of fibrous changes were believed to be histologically normal. The presumed etiologies included oxygen toxicity and/or barotrauma. However, as management strategies have evolved, younger preterm infants have higher survival rates. As a consequence, the clinical picture of BPD, as well the understanding of the pathogenesis of this disease, has changed considerably.

As alluded to earlier, several authors now distinguish between "old" and "new" BPD.[1,17] The essential features of new BPD are alveolar simplification and enlargement, as well as vascular changes. Alveoli retain a saccular appearance; the distal microvasculature is dysmorphic; and capillaries are abnormally distributed and are generally further away from the air surface. Thus, both angiogenesis and alveolarization are altered in patients with BPD. The following discussion focuses on the authors' current understanding of pathogenesis of BPD, including what is known concerning the molecular mechanisms underlying alveolar and vascular dysfunction. As an introduction, the sequence of lung development is briefly reviewed.

OVERVIEW OF LUNG DEVELOPMENT: ALVEOLAR AND VASCULAR DIFFERENTIATION

Lung development spanning 40 weeks of gestation can be divided into five stages: embryonic, pseudoglandular, canalicular, saccular, and alveolar (**Fig. 1**). Midway through gestation (week 20), the conductive airways are almost complete, but alveoli appear only after 32 weeks of gestation. Nonetheless, the period of viability for preterm birth is generally considered to begin after 23 weeks, by which point lung development is transitioning from the cannalicular phase into the saccular phase.

Vascular events are tightly linked to and partly controlled by alveolar development. Two mechanism of capillary growth can be considered: vasculogenesis and angiogenesis. During the early stages of lung growth (spanning the embryonic and pseudoglandular stages), the developing airways serve as a guide for the growth of new blood vessels via vasculogenesis; this process involves the formation of new blood vessels from mesenchymal progenitor cells. By week 17, or the beginning of the cannalicular stage, new blood vessels begin to be formed via angiogenesis, during which existing capillary endothelial cells give rise to new capillaries.

According the revised or new schema of BPD, both vascular and alveolar development appear

Table 1
Definition of bronchopulmonary dysplasia: diagnostic criteria

Gestational Age	<32 Weeks	≥32 Weeks
Time point of assessment	36 weeks PMA or discharge to home, whichever comes first	> 28 d but < 56 d postnasal age or discharge to home, whichever comes first
	Treatment with oxygen > 21% for at least 28 d plus	
Mild BPD	Breathing room air at 36 weeks PMA or discharge, whichever comes first	Breathing room air by 56 d postnatal age or discharge, whichever comes first
Moderate BPD	Need[a] for < 30% oxygen at 36 weeks PMA or discharge, whichever comes first	Need[a] for < 30% oxygen at 56 d postnatal age or discharge, whichever comes first
Severe BPD	Need[a] for ≥ 30% oxygen and/or positive pressure, (PPV or NCPAP) at 36 weeks PMA or discharge, whichever comes first	Need[a] for ≥ 30% oxygen and/or positive pressure (PPV or NCPAP) at 56 d postnatal age or discharge, whichever comes first

Abbreviations: BPD, bronchopulmonary dysplasia; NCPAP, nasal continuous positive airway pressure; PMA, postmenstrual age; PPV, positive-pressure ventilation.
[a] A physiologic test confirming that the oxygen requirement at the assessment time point remains to be defined. This assessment may include a pulse oximetry saturation range. *From* Jobe AH, Bancalari E. Bronchopulmonary dysplasia. Am J Respir Crit Care Med 2001;163(7):1723–9; with permission.

to be impaired, with the level of airway injury and fibrosis either mild or nonexistent. In contrast, in the old model of BPD, the level of alveolar development appeared to be normal in the absence of fibrosis. This difference in presentation between old and ne BPD, which is dependent in part on advances in neonatal care, has lead to a conceptual shift: whereas oxygen toxicity and mechanical

ventilation were considered to be the primary causes of BPD, it is perhaps more useful to consider the cause to be factors which interfere with development.[18] This also shifts the time frame of initial induction of BPD: rather than the focus being on postnatal events, more consideration is given to the period spanning the late cannalicular and early saccular stages of lung development. It is important, then, to discuss some of the factors that modulate this phase of lung development.

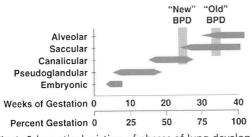

Fig. 1. Schematic depiction of phases of lung development during gestation. Old bronchopulmonary dysplasia (BPD) developed in children who were born in the saccular and alveolar phases. In contrast, new BPD is seen in preterm infants of extremely low gestational age who are born in the canalicular and early saccular phases of lung development. (*From* Kramer BW. Antenatal inflammation and lung injury: prenatal origin of neonatal disease. J Perinatol 2008;28:S21–7; with permission. Copyright © 2008, Nature Publishing Group.)

MODERATORS OF ALVEOLAR AND VASCULAR DEVELOPMENT

In the normal course of prenatal and postnatal lung development, a complex web of factors regulates vascular development and airway differentiation. With the aid of modern molecular techniques, including genetic "knock-out" animal models and RNA silencing, a multitude of transcription factors, bioactive peptides and signaling molecules have been shown to be involved in regulating lung growth and differentiation. Several of the factors, or morphogens, have been shown to be altered in animal and human studies of BPD, thereby providing clues as to the mechanisms and etiologies of BPD.

Vascular endothelial growth factor (VEGF) coordinates epithelial and vascular development, and is required for the development of lung vasculature; in turn, the pulmonary vasculature is necessary for airway epithelial proliferation and morphogenesis.[19–21] A clue suggesting that a vascular dysgenesis may be associated with BDP and delayed alveolarization is the finding that human infants dying with BPD have decreased expression of VEGF and of the angiogenic receptors, Flt-1 and Tie-2, in lung tissue samples (**Fig. 2**).[22] Moreover, these findings may be of clinical significance: Lassus and colleagues[23] determined that infants diagnosed with BPD have lower levels of VEGF in tracheal apirates. They also found that infants with more severe respiratory distress syndrome (RDS) had lower levels of VEGF. Experiments involving rat pups with hyperoxia-induced BPD have shown that genetically-enhanced expression of VEGF can promote lung maturation.[24] These findings suggest that VEGF may potentially used in both diagnosis and treatment of BPD. Still other studies have shown correlations between anti-angiogenic factors and BPD. For example, endothelial–monocyte activrating polypeptide (EMAP) is elevated and abnormally distributed in the lung tissue of an animal model of BPD.[25]

Other factors associated with BPD involve either the lung extracellular matrix or the airway epithelium itself. The extracellular matrix contains not only structural proteins, such as collagen (predominantly collagens I, III and IV), reticulin and elastin. There are also a wide range of attachment factors and morphogens, which together guide and direct both proliferation and differentiation of the lung epithelium. The matrix is also under constant flux. It is continually synthesized and degraded. Two key enzymes involved in maintaining this balance between deposition and destruction are: matrix metalloproteases (MMPs) and tissue inhibitors of MMPs (TIMPs), respectively.

It is beyond the scope of this review to describe the various members of this family of enzymes.[26] In summary: in infants with BPD, there is an increase in collagen deposition in situ; there are also elevated levels of collagen type IV in tracheal aspirates of infants with BPD. Such findings indicate inflammation and basement membrane damage, which can have profound influences on the differentiation of lung tissues. In addition to the more visible signs of increased collagen deposition, either the expression or localization of specific MMPs and TIMPs have been found in children with BPD.[26] These findings correlate well with observed changes in the lung extracellular matrix, although the precise triggers for these changes await further elucidation.

A number of other transcription factors and signal molecules appear to be associated with the pathogenesis of BPD. Another peptide, parathyroid hormone-related protein (PTHrP), which is produced by type II pneumocytes, acts in a paracrine fashion to stimulate the differentiation of new type II cells. In patients who have BPD, there is a deficiency in PTHrP, which is apparently triggered by alveolar overdistension, which in turn

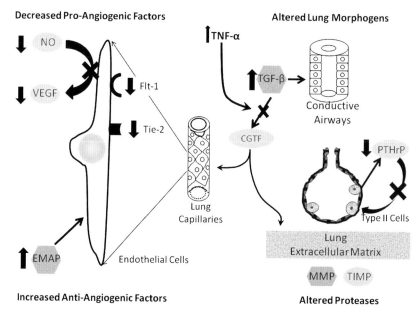

Fig. 2. Schematic depicting decreased expression of VEGF and of the angiogenic receptors, Flt-1 and Tie-2.

has a negative feedback effect on type II cell proliferation and alveolar differentiation.[26] Other peptide signal molecules are also altered in either animal studies of BPD, such as keratinocyte growth factor, gastrin-releasing peptide, and transforming growth factor-beta (TGF-β). The latter inhibits branching of the airways, and in rat studies, TGF-β overexpression induces patchy fibrotic changes.

Although alterations in the above-named growth factors and signals help in the understanding of some of the tissue alteration that occur in patients who have BPD, the pathophysiological basis or "trigger" for their up- or down-regulation needs description. The subsequent section reviews the evidence and the key theories currently proposed for the pathogenesis of BPD.

PRE- AND POSTNATAL ORIGINS OF BPD
Prenatal Factors: Chorioamnionitis

The inflammatory response is a central player in the initiation of BPD. This assertion is corroborated by the presence of many of the classic pro-inflammatory markers in the tracheal aspirates of infants who are diagnosed with BPD. The inflammatory response may be initiated antenatally or postnatally. Although somewhat equivocal, chorioamnionitis was initially associated with BPD by Watterberg and colleagues[27] Conflicting evidence has come from cohort studies by Kent and Dahlstrom[28] and Andrews and colleagues,[29] in which these investigators reported that chorioamnionitis was not associated with BPD. Nevertheless, animal models of chorioamnionitis, primarily using fetal sheep, have been developed that clearly implicate antenatal infection and inflammation in the pathogenesis of BPD. Intra-amniotic injection of endotoxin, a bacterial cell wall product that binds to Toll-like receptors, induces several markers of inflammation in fetal sheep, including monocytes and macrophages in bronchiolar aspirates, and mRNA for the pro-inflammatory cytokines IL-1β, IL-6 and IL-8 in lung tissue.[30]

A number of other indicators of inflammation and lung injury have also been detected in the preterm lamb/sheep model of chorioamnionitis,[18] but, most strikingly, reduced vascular and alveolar development were also noted within 7 days of intra-amniotic injection.[31,32] Furthermore, several mediators of vascular development are also reduced in these lambs, including VEGF and VEGF receptor, platelet endothelial cell adhesion molecule, and connective tissue growth factor (CTGF).[33] TNF-α, another pro-inflammatory cytokine, is also elevated after endotoxin injection, as is TGF-β.[34] Although TGF-β, which is elevated in

this scenario, normally up-regulates CGTF, one theory is that the increased levels of TNF-α inhibit the tropic effect of TGF-β (see **Fig. 2**).[18] Because CGTF is involved in both regulating connective tissue synthesis and in promoting vascular development, these lower levels of CGTF are also consistent with the presentation of BPD.

Although the vascular and alveolar signs of BPD are induced in preterm lambs from dams with chorioamnionitis, the ultimate functional effects of endotoxin injection were increases in lung surfactant, compliance, gas exchange and oxygenation.[18,31] This seeming paradox suggests that endotoxin may, indeed, confer a survival advantage, presumably by up-regulating other factors that eventually promote lung maturation. This would argue for the role of postnatal factors in further promoting and exacerbating the arrested lung development seen in infants with BPD.

From a clinical perspective, pathogens that are likely to be associated with chorioamnionitis (and therefore the incidence of BPD) include mycoplasma or ureaplasma.[35] Further complicating this picture, there is an association between BPD and antenatal steroids. At first inspection this appears to be a paradox: the efficacy of antenatal steroids to induce fetal lung maturation is very well established, and initially betamethasone inhibits the inflammatory response. However, in the fetal sheep model, administration of both endotoxin and steroids resulted in significantly higher levels of inflammatory cells and mediators 5 to 15 days post exposure than did endotoxin alone.[33] A possible explanation is that maternal betamethasone treatments initially suppress, then augment, the inflammatory responses of fetal monocytes. This may be clinically relevant in women who have clinically silent chorioamnionitis and who receive betamethasone. In such instances, steroids may up-regulate inflammatory cells.

Postnatal Factors: Oxidative Stress

It is well established that preterm infants are at particular risk of oxidative stress, which is essentially an imbalance between antioxidant defenses (eg, catalases, glutathione peroxidases, and superoxide dismutase) and reactive oxygen species (ROS), such as hydroxyl and superoxide anions, hydrogen peroxide and peroxynitrates. At birth, the preterm infant has lower catalase,[36] cysteine (a precursor of glutathione)[37] and other antioxidants; coupled with neonatal exposure to high oxygen tensions during resuscitation or supplemental oxygen therapy, the risk of oxidative stress is particularly high. Where this fits in with BPD is that oxidative stress regulates an extensive array of antioxidant response element (ARE)-driven genes, which, in turn, code for protein products that are involved in inflammation, cell signaling, and alveolar development, to name a few. Attempts to minimize oxidative stress by providing exogenous antioxidants may, therefore, meet with some success in reducing the morbidity and/or incidence of BPD. This work is complicated by the fact that any such interventions would need to occur before ARE genes are activated. Alternately, oxidative stress levels may be reduced by minimizing the level of exposure to high oxygen partial pressures, although this has not yet been clinically shown to improve BOD outcomes.

Postnatal Factors: Mechanical Ventilation

Lung injury secondary to resuscitation and/or ventilatory support are life-saving interventions that come with a cost. Lung damage can be accrued either through inadequate positive end expiratory pressures (and subsequent alveolar collapse) or through hyperinflation and barotrauma.[35] Mechanically-ventilated preterm infants chronically develop inflammation, with a cascade of inflammatory cytokines associated with higher incidence and severity of BPD, and they also have significant surfactant dysfunction. Although the use of exogenous surfactant has greatly ameliorated lung damage, it is still far from clear what are the optimal ventilatory strategies.[35]

Postnatal Factors and BPD: Nutrition

In a general sense, adequate nutrition is important for optimal postnatal development. However, the question as to whether poor nutrition exacerbates BPD is still open. Preterm infants have, for example, lower N-acetylcysteine, vitamins A and E, and inositol levels, all of which may impact either antioxidant protection, lung development and/or surfactant production.[26] It is still unclear whether interventions aimed at supplementing preterm infants have a significant impact on the incidence of BOD.

Chessex and colleagues[38] have recently promulgated an interesting hypothesis: that development of BPD is influenced by lipid peroxidation in total parenteral nutrition (TPN). TPN is usually given to preterm infants until full enteral nutrition is established, although this does come with some possible complications, for example, failure to shield TPN generates lipid peroxides, which in turn add to oxidant stress in the neonate[39,40] and to lung remodeling.[39] The work of Chessex and colleagues has provided preliminary evidence that photoprotection of TPN is associated with a 30% decrease in BPD in human infants. This study paves the way for future multicenter trials that, if confirmatory of the original hypothesis, will support the implementation of a simple intervention – light-shielding TPN, which may significantly reduce the morbidity and mortality of BPD.

PREVENTATIVE STRATEGIES

Because BPD is a disease the primarily affects premature neonates, the optimal strategy for preventing BPD is to prevent preterm birth. Given that 69% of preterm singleton births occur spontaneously and 31% occur for medical indications,[41] prevention is not always possible. When preterm delivery cannot be prevented, antenatal steroids should be administered. The effectiveness of antenatal steroids in reducing the severity of RDS and need for respiratory report has been well established in numerous research studies as well as the Cochrane review of these studies.[42] Further, a 2008 review[43] of current science done by the American Academy of Pediatrics' Committee on the Fetus and Newborn identifies that antenatal steroids combined with postnatal surfactant work synergistically to reduce the severity of RDS, air leaks, and mortality in premature infants.

Although some measures used to prevent premature infants from developing BPD have been investigated, few have been proven to be effective. In 2003, a group of nine hospitals from the Neonatal Intensive Care Quality Collaborative (NIQ/2000) developed a list of potentially better practices aimed at reducing the incidence and severity of BPD in low birth weight infants.[44] The identified practices include: Vitamin A supplementation; decreased fluid administration; postextubation continuous positive airway pressure (CPAP); permissive hypercarbia; decreased exposure to high-dose corticosteroids; prophylactic surfactant or delivery room CPAP for infants <1000 g; avoiding ventilation or reducing the number of ventilator days; high-frequency or low tidal volume ventilation; and gentle ventilation in the delivery room. The evidence supporting selected practices is reviewed here.

Vitamin A

The administration of vitamin A is one of the only measures that has been definitively shown to affect the development of BPD.[45] A Cochrane review of vitamin A for the prevention of BPD found that this drug was effective in reducing the rate of oxygen dependency at 36 weeks gestation.[46]

Although there is level I evidence supporting the use of vitamin A, a survey conducted in 2003 found that only 20% of teaching NICUs and 13% of non-teaching units were routinely giving vitamin A to LBW infants.[47]

The role of several other antioxidant agents in the prevention of BPD has been investigated, such as, intratracheal superoxide dismutase[48] and n-acetylcysteine.[49] Neither agent resulted in any significant improvement in BPD rates.

Fluid Restriction

Pulmonary edema has been shown to result from lung injury and inflammation. The presence of excessive lung water has been linked to the development of BPD.[50] Because of the relationship between lung water and BPD, it is recommended that fluid intake in LWB infants be restricted to the minimum necessary to provide adequate calories for growth.[51,52] In a meta-analysis Bell and Acarregui[53] demonstrated that, in premature infants, restricted fluid intake results in lower mortality and a trend toward a lower incidence of BPD.

Prophylactic Surfactant

The benefits of exogenous surfactant in reducing the severity of RDS and increasing survival in the LBW infant have been established by numerous randomized controlled trials (RCTs) and systematic reviews.[54–58] Despite the reduction in initial oxygen and ventilatory requirements, the incidence of BPD in ELBW neonates has not changed with surfactant replacement; however, the number of ELBW infants who are surviving without BPD has increased.[59,60]

A recent Cochrane analysis found that when the early use of surfactant is combined with extubation to nasal continuous positive airway pressure (NCPAP), there are these results: less need for mechanical ventilation; fewer air leaks; and a lower rate of BPD than in infants receiving surfactant later.[61] The reduction in BPD was also increased when surfactant treatment was given when FiO_2 at study entry was <0.45 rather than >0.45.

Avoiding Mechanical Ventilation/Lung Protective Ventilation

The link between mechanical ventilation and the development of CLD has been clearly established.[13,62] What is less clear is which component or combination of components of ventilation (ie, pressure, volume or oxygen) is of greatest concern. It seems most likely that a combination of these factors, in addition to acute lung injury caused by inflammation, surfactant deficiency and other yet-to-be identified etiologies, is responsible for the development of BPD.

Given the contribution of mechanical ventilation to lung injury, it is not surprising that a great deal of attention has been given to finding less harmful ways to support premature infants with respiratory disease. There are several approaches to achieve the goal of reducing neonatal exposure to injurious ventilation strategies: gentle ventilation during resuscitation; the avoidance of ventilation by using CPAP; brief intubation with surfactant administration followed by extubation to CPAP; and less aggressive approaches to mechanical ventilation including synchronized ventilation and high frequency ventilation. None of these strategies have been shown to prevent BPD, but some reduction in the incidence and severity of BPD has been seen.[45]

Results of research comparing the efficacy of various devices and approaches to ventilation have been mixed. Many of the studies suffer from small numbers, as well as from varied definitions and protocols. Meta-analyses are difficult because of changes in practice that occur over time. For example, many of the CPAP and high frequency ventilation studies took place before the generalized use of antenatal steroids and surfactant. Multicenter studies are important in achieving larger sample sizes, but such studies are confounded by local approaches to care that make controlling variables difficult. Finally, many of the studies have used conventional mechanical ventilation for the comparison group. With the advent of newer synchronized modes of ventilation, this comparison may not be valid.[63] These approaches are reviewed below.

Gentle Ventilation in the Delivery Room

The premature neonate's lung is highly susceptible to injury and, when injured, the lung responds with an exaggerated inflammatory response.[64] Seminal research done by Bjorklund and colleagues[65] demonstrated that, in lambs, ventilation with as few as six manual breaths with 35–40 mL/kg before surfactant administration diminished the alveolar response to subsequent surfactant administration. The lungs of the bagged lambs were more difficult to ventilate and showed more evidence of tissue damage than control lambs. Further animal research has demonstrated that initial resuscitation with high tidal volumes increases both lung edema[66–68] and the production of inflammatory cytokines[68] resulting in decreased surfactant production.[69] This work supports the findings of Hussey, and colleagues[70] who recommend that devices used for manual ventilation in very low birth weight (VLBW) infants be equipped with manometers and positive end expiratory pressure (PEEP) valves.

Use of Nasal CPAP

The noninvasive nature of CPAP suggests that it should provide a more gentle approach to respiratory support, possibly reducing the neonate's exposure to the damaging effects of pressure and volume, which are associated with mechanical ventilation. Despite this assumption, research results have been mixed.[63,71]

Similarly to other areas of neonatal research, many of the studies examining NPAP took place before the introduction of surfactant.[72] This problem makes the interpretation of the data more difficult. Animal research comparing 2 hours of CPAP or continuous mandatory ventilation (CMV) immediately after birth demonstrated that those animals on CPAP had higher lung volumes and less evidence of inflammatory changes compared with animals receiving CMV.[73] The use of NCPAP[74] or rapid shallow ventilation rather than slow deep breaths[75] in animal models has also been shown to improve the development of lung alveoli.[75]

Studies of premature infants older than 27 weeks' gestation have shown that early use of CPAP may lessen the incidence of BPD.[6,13,76] In one of the early publications on the subject, Avery and colleagues[6] compared rates of BPD at eight United States' NICUs. They found that the incidence of BPD was significantly lower at one center, Columbia Presbyterian Medical Center in New York, than at others. Further analysis of the data pointed to Columbia's early use of nasal prong CPAP and lower rates of mechanical ventilation as the most likely reasons for the difference. This conclusion was similar to the findings in a more recent study done by Van Marter and colleagues[13] comparing BPD rates and care practices at three large United States' NICUs. Results showed a significantly higher rate of BPD in two of the hospitals compared with the third. When care practices were analyzed, the most significant difference between the units with higher BPD rates compared with the unit with the lower rate was the percentage of infants receiving mechanical ventilation (75% vs. 29%).

An RCT of 207 premature infants assigned infants to either early or rescue CPAP; the study found a significant reduction in BPD in the early CPAP group.[77] Of note, bag and mask ventilation with initial pressure of 30–40 cm water pressure was used for some infants in the control group, while infants in the early CPAP group received a sustained inflation of 20 cm water pressure at the time of birth. It could be speculated that the initial breaths with large inflation pressures in the control group may have played a result in the findings.[63] In a retrospective study of bubble CPAP done in New Zealand, Meyer and colleagues[78] identified an CLD rate of 19% compared with an average of 45% in 28 other centers. Other studies have confirmed the benefit of using prophylactic CPAP.[79,80]

In contrast, a RCT of 610 infants born between 25 and 28 weeks gestation concluded that nasal CPAP applied within 5 minutes of birth did not significantly reduce the incidence of BPD when compared with intubation.[81] Similarly, in a study of 230 infants 28–31 weeks gestation, Sandri and colleagues[72] compared the prophylactic use of CPAP with CPAP applied when the infant's FIO_2 requirement reached 40% and they did not find a significant difference in the need for mechanical ventilation or in long-term outcomes. The CPAP group did have a higher incidence of pneumothorax, but the patients had fewer days of ventilation. A meta-analysis examining prophylactic CPAP showed no significant differences in BPD rates.[82] However, this analysis included only two trials, one of which used nasopharyngeal CPAP and the other using nasal prong CPAP. In one of the studies, no antenatal steroids were used; in the other study, only 20%–25% of the infants in the CPAP or control groups received surfactant.

A newer approach to the use of nasal CPAP in VLBW infants, dubbed the "INSURE" approach, involves intubation and administration of surfactant, followed by rapid extubation to CPAP.[83] The use of this approach in one center in Sweden reduced the number of neonates needing mechanical ventilation by 50%.[83] In a retrospective study of infants less than 27 weeks, 14 of 21 infants extubated on the first day of life remained successfully extubated.[84] A meta-analysis of six studies using this approach found a significant reduction in BPD in the infants extubated early to CPAP.[61] Of note, more infants in the early extubation arm of these trials received surfactant and also received a greater number of doses of surfactant, a factor which may influence the outcome.[63]

Variable flow CPAP or nasal positive pressure ventilation (NIPPV), recently introduced, provides an additional level of respiratory support without the complications of intubation and mechanical ventilation. Early research into this mode of noninvasive ventilation suggests that it may be of greater benefit than conventional CPAP in reducing CLD. Courtney and colleagues[85] evaluated 32 infants weighing <1800 g and found that lung recruitment was improved in the variable flow infants compared with those receiving continuous flow CPAP. In an RCT evaluating NIPPV, a trend toward lower rates of BPD was noted but the numbers did not reach statistical significance.[86] A recent study[87] found that in the 84 infants 28–33 weeks in their study, those randomized to NIPPV for the initial treatment of RDS were significantly less likely to require ventilation than those in the CPAP group (25% vs. 49%) and had significantly lower rates of BPD (5% vs. 33%, $P < .05$, for infants <1500 g).

Despite conflicting results from research studies, it is clear that nasal CPAP is a useful mode of support for reducing the need for mechanical ventilation. In a summary of the science on surfactant and CPAP, the American Academy of Pediatrics Committee on the Fetus and Newborn[43] concluded that CPAP, with or without surfactant administration may reduce the incidence of BPD. They point out, however, that no large RCTs have been done to validate this conclusion.

Post-Extubation CPAP

The use of CPAP following extubation reduces the need for re-intubation and therefore helps to reduce the infant's exposure to mechanical ventilation.[88] Questions remain regarding the optimal levels of CPAP and the gestational age at which most benefit is attained.

Permissive Hypercarbia

Allowing elevated levels of $PaCO_2$[45–55] has been suggested as another way to avoid aggressive ventilation. By allowing higher levels of carbon dioxide, the need for higher pressures with resulting baro- and volutrauma is reduced.[89,90] Retrospective studies have demonstrated a lower incidence of BPD in infants whose PCO_2 was maintained at a higher level in the first four days of life.[91–93] A randomized controlled trial of 49 preterm infants weighing between 601 and 1200 g conducted by Carlo and colleagues[94] demonstrated that mild elevations in pO_2 (45–55 mm HG) resulted in a significant reduction in the duration of mechanical ventilation, 2.5 days compared with 9.5 days in the control group. On the other hand, a Cochrane review found no evidence that permissive hypercapnia reduced the incidence of death or CLD at 36 weeks.[95]

High Frequency Ventilation

High-frequency ventilation (HFV) uses rapid rates and small tidal volumes to deliver gases to the alveoli. Animal studies have shown a promising reduction in airway injury and CLD with the use of HFV.[96–103] Data from premature infants has been less convincing. Many of the studies of HFV were done before the use of antenatal steroids or surfactant and many studies have suffered from small numbers and inconsistent protocols.

A key to successful treatment with high-frequency ventilation is maintaining adequate lung volumes and functional residual capacity;[104,105] however, many HFV studies have used low mean airway pressures, which may be to blame for a failure to demonstrate a reduction in BPD.[106] In 2002, two large randomized trial of high-frequency oscillatory ventilation (HFOV) were reported. One study[107] found that in infants of 500–1200 g, survival without CLD was 56% in the HFOV group compared with 47% in the conventional ventilation group, while the other study[108] found no significant difference in survival or CLD in 787 infant between 23 and 28 weeks of gestation.

A meta-analysis of 16 RCTS and four systematic reviews done by van Kaam and Rimensberger[109] noted that there were no consistent differences found in BPD rates or mortality in their review. They commented that a number of studies in their analysis suffered from design weaknesses. In particular, some RCTs did not randomize patients for several hours after birth and others had a high rate of crossover between HFV and CMV. In some studies it was unclear what percentage of patients were exposed to antenatal steroids or surfactant; studies differed in the gestational ages of infants included.[109]

A Cochrane Review[110] of 11 RCTS done between 1989 and 2003 found no difference in mortality rates at 28 days or at 36 weeks postmenstrual age. Three trials in this review demonstrated a decreased risk of CLD at 36 weeks.[107,111,112] In the combined analysis, there was a decrease in the risk of CLD or death at 36 or 37 weeks.

In a 2007 update of their previous Cochrane review, Henderson-Smart and colleagues[113] included 15 studies of HFOV with a total enrollment of 3585 infants. However, the results of the analysis did not change significantly. There continues to be no significant difference in mortality rates at 28–30 days of age or at 36–37 weeks, despite a small decrease in the rates of CLD with HFOV.

Bhuta and colleagues[114] reviewed high-frequency jet ventilation (HFJV) for both initial and rescue[115] treatment of preterm infants with RDS. The incidence of CLD was no different with HFJV than with CMV at 28 days, but one study[116] did find a decrease in CLD at 36 weeks in infants receiving HFJV.

The availability of newer synchronized ventilators capable of targeting volumes and concerns about the potential for hyperventilation and subsequent neurologic injury continues to cause hesitation in the use of HFV as an initial strategy for ventilating the premature infant with RDS.[113,117]

Lung Protective Ventilation

Over the past 15 years, ventilator technology has improved greatly. More sensitive monitoring devices have been developed that allow all but the smallest infants to trigger ventilator breaths. This allows ventilator breaths to be delivered in synchrony with the infant's breath. In addition, pressure support and volume-targeted modes of ventilation have been developed that provide additional options for the clinician attempting to avoid lung damage in the VLBW infant.

In a study comparing synchronous intermittent mandatory ventilation (SIMV) with conventional nonsynchronized ventilation for infant <1000 g, Bernstein and colleagues[118] found that SIMV-treated neonates had a lower incidence of BPD than those on conventional ventilation. Other RCTs have shown that synchronization facilitated weaning, leading to a reduction in ventilator day but did not show consistent reduction in BPD rates.[119–123] Again, there were a number of important differences across these trials that may have affected the results including: postmenstrual age, age at randomization, a high rate of crossover to other modes of ventilation, and problems with the sensitivity of the triggering device in some studies.[124] A meta-analysis by Greenough and colleagues[125] concurred that triggered ventilation was not associated with a significant decrease in BPD.

A review of the current literature done by van Kaam and Rimensberger[109] found 24 RCTs and three systematic reviews that compared various types modes of CMV and various ventilator strategies. They also reviewed two RCTs that examined permissive hypercapnia in infants at risk for BPD. Their review demonstrated no differences in BPD rates or in mortality, however, they point out that no RCTs examined different tidal volumes or levels of PEEP, variables that may be critical in preventing lung injury. Failure to use enough PEEP to maintain adequate levels of end expiratory lung volume results in collapse of the alveoli and small airways (atelectrauma).[126]

Given the relationship between alveolar overdistension or alveolar collapse (atelectrauma) and acute lung injury[127] it is important to pay particular attention to the ventilator strategies being used in an attempt to prevent CLD. It may be that failure to employ a strategy that recruits and maintains the volume in the alveoli (open lung strategy) will offset the benefits gained by other protective strategies, such as synchronized or volume targeted ventilation.[109] Aminal studies have demonstrated that using an open lung strategy may be more important than limiting lung volumes or preventing atelectasis alone.[128] Further research is needed to carefully examine ventilator strategies to optimize lung protection.

SUMMARY

The etiology of BPD involves the complex interplay of a number of genetic, environmental, and individual factors. A thorough understanding of the pathogenesis of BPD is critical in developing appropriate care practices to minimize lung injury in the VLBW infant. An appreciation of the impact of even small changes in ventilation, nutritional practices, and fluid administration highlights the need to develop a comprehensive multidisciplinary approach to care of these infants. Although our understanding of the importance of fluids and nutrition, antioxidants, and ventilation strategies has grown markedly in the past ten years, many questions remain. Clearly further large-scale, multicentered trials are needed to answer remaining questions. While awaiting results from such trials, it is important that to continue to examine best practices and to use benchmarking data to evaluate the success of centers with low rates of BPD to better understand which strategies are most successful in minimizing the long-term respiratory morbidities associated with prematurity.

REFERENCES

1. Coalson JJ. Pathology of bronchopulmonary dysplasia. Semin Perinatol 2006;30(4):179–84.
2. Bhandari A, Panitch HB. Pulmonary outcomes in bronchopulmonary dysplasia. Semin Perinatol 2006;30(4):219–26.
3. Northway WH, Rosan RC, Porter DY. Pulmonary disease following respirator therapy of hyaline membrane disease: bronchopulmonary dysplasia. N Engl J Med 1967;276(7):357–68.
4. Bancalari E, Abdenour GE, Feller R, et al. Bronchopulmonary dysplasia: clinical presentation. J Pediatr 1979;95(5 part 2):819–23.
5. Bancalari E, Claure N. Definitions and diagnostic criteria for bronchopulmonary dysplasia. Semin Perinatol 2006;30(4):164–70.
6. Avery ME, Tooley WH, Keller JB, et al. Is chronic lung disease in low birth weight infants preventable? A survey of eight centers. Pediatrics 1987; 79(1):26–30.
7. Sinkin RA, Cox C, Phelps DL. Predicting risk for bronchopulmonary dysplasia: selection criteria for clinical trials. Pediatrics 1990;86(5):728–36.
8. Shennan AT, Dunn MS, Ohlsson A, et al. Abnormal pulmonary outcomes in premature infants: prediction from oxygen requirement in the neonatal period. Pediatrics 1988;82(4):527–32.
9. Palta M, Sadek M, Barnet JH, et al. Evaluation of criteria for chronic lung disease in surviving very low birthweight infants. Newborn Lung Project. J Pediatr 1998;132(1):57–63.
10. Jobe AH, Bancalari E. Bronchopulmonary dysplasia. Am J Respir Crit Care Med 2001;163(7):1723–9.

11. Jobe AH, Bancalari E. Workshop on bronchopul-monary dysplasia National Institutes of Health. Available at: http://rarediseases.info.nih.gov/asp/html/conferences/conferences/Broncho20000601.htm. 2000 [accessed July 15 2008].

12. Davis JM, Rosenfeld WN. Bronchopulmonary dysplasia. In: MacDonald MG, Mullett MD, Seshia MMK, editors. Avery's neonatology. Pathophysiology and management of the newborn. 6th edition. Philadelphia: Lippincott Williams & Wilkins; 2005. p. 578–99.

13. Van Marter LJ, Allred EN, Pagano M, et al. Do clinical markers of barotrauma and oxygen toxicity explain interhospital variation in rates of chronic lung disease? Pediatrics 2000;105:1194–201.

14. Walsh MC, Yao Q, Gettner P, et al. Impact of a physiologic definition on bronchopulmonary dysplasia rates. Pediatrics 2004;114(5):1305–11.

15. Sahni R, Ammari A, Suri MS, et al. Is the new definition of bronchopulmonary dysplasia more useful? J Perinatol 2005;25:41–6.

16. Ehrenkranz RA, Walsh MC, Vohr BR, et al. National Institutes of child health and human development neonatal research network. Validation of the National Institutes of Health consensus definition of bronchopulmonary dysplasia. Pediatrics 2005; 116(6):1353–60.

17. Jobe AH. The new BPD. Neoreviews 2008;7(10): e531–43.

18. Kramer BW. Antenatal inflammation and lung injury: prenatal origin of neonatal disease. J Pernatol 2008;28:S21–7.

19. Zhao L, Wang K, Ferrara N, et al. Vascular endothelial growth factor co-ordinates proper development of lung epithelium and vasculature. Mech Dev 2005;122(7–8):877–86.

20. Jakkula M, Le Cras TD, Gebb S, et al. Inhibition of angiogenesis decreases alveolarization the developing rat lung. Am J Physiol Lung Cell Mol Physiol 2000;279:L600–7.

21. Maniscalco WM, Watkins RH, Pyhruber GS, et al. Angeogenic factors and alveolar vasculature: development and alterations by injury in very premature baboons. Am J Physiol Lung Cell Mol Physiol 2002;282:L811–23.

22. Bhatt AJ, Pryhuber GS, Huyck H, et al. Disrupted pulmonary vasculature and decreased vascular endothelial growth factor, Flt-1, and Tie-2 in human infants dying with bronchopulmonary dysplasia. Am J Respir Crit Care Med 2001;164:1971–80.

23. Lassus P, Ristimäki A, Ylikorkala O, et al. Vascular endothelial growth factor in human preterm lung. Am J Respir Crit Care Med 1999;159(5 Pt 1): 1429–33.

24. Thebaud B, Ladha F, Michelakis E, et al. Vascular endothelial growth factor gene therapy increases survival, promotes lung angiogenesis, and prevents alveolar damage in hyperoxia-induced lung injury: evidence that angiogenesis participates in alveolarization. Circulation 2005;112(16): 2477–86.

25. Quintos-Alagheband ML, White CW, Schwarz MA. Potential role for antiangiogenic proteins in the evolution of bronchopulmonary dysplasia. Antioxid Redox Signal 2004;6(1):137–45.

26. Ambavalam N, Carlo WA. Bronchopulmonary dysplasia: new insights. Clin Perinatol 2004;31:613–28.

27. Watterberg KL, Demers LM, Scott SM, et al. Chorioamnionitis and early lung inflammation in infants in whom bronchopulmonary dysplasia develops. Pediatrics 1996;97(2):210–5.

28. Kent A, Dahlstrom JE. Chorioamnitis/funisitis and the development of bronchopulmonary dysplasia. J Pediatr Child Health 2004;40:356–9.

29. Andrews WW, Goldberg RI, Faye-Petersen O, et al. The Alabama Preterm Birth Study: polymorphonuclear and mononuclear cell placental infiltrations, other markers of inflammation, and outcomes in 23- to 32-week preterm newborn infants. Am J Obstet Gynecol 2006;195:803–8.

30. Kramer BW, Kaemmerer U, Kapp M, et al. Decreased expression of angiogenic factors in placentas with chorioamnitis after preterm birth. Pediatr Res 2005;58:607–12.

31. Jobe AH, Newnham JP, Wilet KE, et al. Effects of antenatal endotoxin on the lungs of preterm lambs. Am J Obstet Gynecol 2000;182:401–8.

32. Willet KE, Jobe AH, Ikegami M, et al. Antenatal endotoxin and glucocorticoid effects on lung morphometry in preterm lambs. Pediatr Res 2000; 48:782–8.

33. Kallipur SG, Bachurski CJ, Le Cras TD, et al. Vascular changes after intra-amniotic endotoxin in preterm lamb lungs. Am J Physiol Lung Cell Mol Physiol 2004;287:L1178–85.

34. Kunzman S, Speer CP, Jobe AH, et al. Antenatal inflammation induced TGF-{beta}1 but suppressed CTGF in preterm lungs. Am J Physiol Lung Cell Mol Physiol 2007;292:L223–31.

35. Chess PR, D'Agnio CT, Pryhuber GS, et al. Pathogenesis of bronchopulmonary dysplasia. Semin Perinatol 2006;30:171–8.

36. Asikainen TM, Raivio KO, Saksela M, et al. Expression and developmental profile of antioxidant enzymes in human lung and liver. Am J Respirol Cell Mol Physiol 1998;19:942–9.

37. Jain A, Mehta T, Auld PA, et al. Glutathione metabolism in newborns: evidence for glutathione deficiency in plasma, broncheoalveolar lavage fluid and lymphocytes in prematures. Pediatr Pulmonol 1995;20:160–6.

38. Chessex P, Harrison A, Khashu M, et al. In preterm neonates, the risk of developing bronchopulmonary dysplasia influenced by the failure to protect

total parenteral nutrition from exposure to ambient light? J Pediatr 2007;151:213–4.

39. Lavoie JC, Rouleau T, Gagnon C, et al. Photoprotection prevents TPN-induced fibrosis in newborn guinea pigs. Free Radic Biol Med 2002;33:512–20.

40. Silvers KM, Sluis KB, Darlow BA, et al. Limiting light-induced lipid peroxidation and vitamin los in infant parenteral nutrition by adding multivitamin preparations to intralipid. Acta Pediatr 2001;90: 242–9.

41. Ananth CV, Joseph KS, Oyelese Y, et al. Trends in preterm birth and perinatal mortality among singletons: United States, 1989 through 2000. Obstet Gynecol 2005;105:1084–91.

42. Roberts D, Dalziel S. Antenatal corticosteroids for accelerating fetal lung maturation for women at risk of preterm birth. Cochrane Database Syst Rev 2006;3:CD004454.

43. Engle WA. American academy of pediatrics committee on fetus and newborn. Surfactant-replacement therapy for respiratory distress in the preterm and term neonate. Pediatrics 2008; 121(2):419–32.

44. Sharek PJ, Baker R, Litman F, et al. Evaluation and development of potentially better practices to prevent chronic lung disease and reduce lung injury in neonates. Pediatrics 2003;111:e426–31.

45. Van Marter LJ. Strategies for preventing bronchopulmonary dysplasia. Curr Opin Pediatr 2005; 17(2):174–80.

46. Darlow BA, Graham PJ. Vitamin A supplementation for preventing morbidity and mortality in very low birthweight infants. Cochrane Database Syst Rev 2002;(4):CD000501.

47. Ambalavanan N, Wu TJ, Tyson JE, et al. A comparison of three vitamin A dosing regimens in extremely-low-birth-weight infants. J Pediatr 2003; 142(6):656–61.

48. Davis JM, Parad RB, Michele T, et al. North American Recombinant Human CuZnSOD Study Group. Pulmonary outcome at 1 year corrected age in premature infants treated at birth with recombinant human CuZn superoxide dismutase. Pediatrics 2003; 111(3):469–76.

49. Ahola T, Lapatto R, Raivio KO, et al. N-acetylcysteine does not prevent bronchopulmonary dysplasia in immature infants:a randomized controlled trial. J Pediatr 2003;143(6):697–8.

50. Adams EW, Harrison MC, Counsell SJ, et al. Increased lung water and tissue damage in bronchopulmonary dysplasia. J Pediatr 2004;145(4): 503–7.

51. Bancalari E. Changes in the pathogenesis and prevention of chronic lung disease of prematurity. Am J Perinatol 2001;18(1):1–9.

52. Oh W, Poindexter BB, Perritt R, et al. Neonatal Research Network. Association between fluid intake and weight loss during the first ten days of life and risk of bronchopulmonary dysplasia in extremely low birth weight infants. J Pediatr 2005; 147(6):786–90.

53. Bell EF, Acarregui MJ. Restricted versus liberal water intake for preventing morbidity and mortality in preterm infants. Cochrane Database Syst Rev 2008;1:CD000503.

54. Yost CC, Soll RF. Early versus delayed selective surfactant treatment for neonatal respiratory distress syndrome. Cochrane Database Syst Rev 2000;1:CD001456.

55. Soll RF, Morley CJ. Prophylactic versus selective use of surfactant in preventing morbidity and mortality in preterm infants. Cochrane Database Syst Rev 2001;2:CD000510.

56. Soll RF. Synthetic surfactant for respiratory distress syndrome in preterm infants. Cochrane Database Syst Rev 2000a;2:CD001149.

57. Soll RF. Prophylactic natural surfactant extract for preventing morbidity and mortality in preterm infants. Cochrane Database Syst Rev 2000b;2: CD000511.

58. Pfister RH, Soll RF, Wiswell T. Protein containing synthetic surfactant versus animal derived surfactant extract for the prevention and treatment of respiratory distress syndrome. Cochrane Database Syst Rev 2007;17(4):CD006069.

59. Yoder BA, Anwar MU, Clark RH. Early prediction of neonatal chronic lung disease: a comparison of three scoring methods. Pediatr Pulmonol 1999;27: 388–94.

60. Jobe AH, Ikegami M. Mechanisms initiating lung injury in the preterm. Early Hum Dev 1998;53:81–94.

61. Stevens TP, Harrington EW, Blennow M, et al. Early surfactant administration with brief ventilation vs. selective surfactant and continued mechanical ventilation for preterm infants with or at risk for respiratory distress syndrome. Cochrane Database Syst Rev 2007;4:CD003063.

62. Clark RH, Gerstmann DR, Jobe AH, et al. Lung injury in neonates: causes, strategies for prevention, and long-term consequences. J Pediatr 2001; 139(4):478–86.

63. Patel DS, Greenough A. Does nasal CPAP reduce bronchopulmonary dysplasia (BPD)? Acta Paediatr; 2008 [published prior to print]. Available at: http://www3.interscience.wiley.com/journal/120835957/abstract [accessed August 2 2008].

64. O'Brodovich HM, Mellins RB. Bronchopulmonary dysplasia. Unresolved neonatal acute lung injury. Am Rev Respir Dis 1985;132:694–709.

65. Bjorklund LJ, Ingimarsson J, Curstedt T, et al. Manual ventilation with a few large breaths at birth compromises the therapeutic effect of subsequent surfactant replacement in immature lambs. Pediatr Res 1997;42:348–55.

66. Carlton DP, Cummings JJ, Scheerer RG, et al. Lung overexpansion increases pulmonary microvascular protein permeability in young lambs. J Appl Phys 1990;69:577–83.

67. Ikegami M, Rebello CM, Jobe AH. Surfactant inhibition by plasma: gestational age and surfactant treatment effects in preterm lambs. J Appl Phys 1996;81:2517–22.

68. Ikegami M, Kallapur S, Michna J, et al. Lung injury and surfactant metabolism after hyperventilation of premature lambs. Pediatr Res 2000;47:398–404.

69. Wada K, Jobe AH, Ikegami M. Tidal volume effects on surfactant treatment responses with the initiation of ventilation in preterm lambs. J Appl Phys 1997; 83:1054–61.

70. Hussey SG, Ryan CA, Murphy BP. Comparison of three manual ventilation devices using an intubated mannequin. Arch Dis Child Fetal Neonatal Ed 2004; 89(6):F490–3.

71. Verder H. Nasal CPAP has become an indispensable part of the primary treatment of newborns with respiratory distress syndrome. Acta Paediatr 2007;96:482–4.

72. Sandri F, Ancora G, Lanzoni A, et al. Prophylactic nasal continuous positive airways pressure in newborns 28–31 weeks gestation: multicenter randomized controlled clinical trial. Arch Dis Child Fetal Neonatal Ed 2004;89(5):F394–8.

73. Jobe AH, Kramer BW, Moss TJ, et al. Decreased indicators of lung injury with continuous positive expiratory pressure in preterm lambs. Pediatr Res 2002;52:387–92.

74. Thomson MA, Yoder BA, Winter VT, et al. Treatment of immature baboons for 28 days with early nasal continuous positive airway pressure. Am J Respir Crit Care Med 2004;169:1054–62.

75. Albertine KH, Jones GP, Starcher BC, et al. Chronic lung injury in preterm lambs. Disordered respiratory tract development. Am J Respir Crit Care Med 1999;159:945–58.

76. Johansson B, Katz-Salamon M, Faxelius G, et al. Neonatal care of very-low-birth weight infants in special-care units and neonatal intensive-care units in Stockholm: early nasal continuous positive airway pressure versus mechanical ventilation—gains and losses. Acta Paediatr Suppl 1997;419:4–10.

77. Te Pas AB, Walthers FJ. A randomised controlled trial of delivery room respiratory management in very preterm infants. Pediatrics 2007;120:322–9.

78. Meyer M, Mildenhall L, Wong M. Outcomes for infants weighing less than 1000 grams cared for with a nasal continuous positive airway pressure–based strategy. J Pediatr Child Health 2004; 40(1–2):38–41.

79. Jacobsen T, Gronvall J, Petersen S, et al. "Minitouch" treatment of very low-birth-weight infants. Acta Paediatr 1993;82:934–8.

80. Gittermann MK, Fusch C, Gittermann AR, et al. Early nasal continuous positive airway pressure treatment reduces the need for intubation in very low birth weight infants. Eur J Pediatr 1997;156: 384–8.

81. Morley CJ, Davis PG, Doyle LW, et al. COIN Trial Investigators. Nasal CPAP or intubation at birth for very preterm infants. N Engl J Med 2008;358(7): 700–8.

82. Subramanian P, Henderson-Smart DJ, Davis PG. Prophylactic nasal continuous positive airway pressure for preventing morbidity and mortality in very preterm infants. Cochrane Database Syst Rev 2005;3:CD001243.

83. Bohlin K, Gudmundsdottir T, Katz-Salamon M, et al. Implementation of surfactant treatment during continuous positive airway pressure. J Perinatol 2007; 27(7):422–7.

84. Booth C, Premkumar MH, Yannoulis A, et al. Sustainable use of continuous positive airway pressure in extremely preterm infants during the first week after delivery. Arch Dis Child Fetal Neonatal Ed 2006;91(6):F398–402.

85. Courtney SE, Pyon KH, Saslow JG, et al. Lung recruitment and breathing pattern during variable versus continuous flow nasal continuous positive airway pressure in premature infants: an evaluation of three devices. Pediatrics 2001;107(2):304–8.

86. Barrington KJ, Bull D, Finer NN. Randomized trial of nasal synchronized intermittent mandatory ventilation compared with continuous positive airway pressure after extubation of very low birth weight infants. Pediatrics 2001;107(4):638–41.

87. Kugelman A, Feferkorn I, Riskin A, et al. Nasal intermittent mandatory ventilation versus nasal continuous positive airway pressure for respiratory distress syndrome: a randomized, controlled, prospective study. J Pediatr 2007;150(5):521–6.

88. Davis PG, Henderson-Smart DJ. Nasal continuous positive airways pressure immediately after extubation for preventing morbidity in preterm infants. Cochrane Database Syst Rev 2003;2:CD000143.

89. Ambalavanan N, Carlo WA. Ventilatory strategies in the prevention and management of bronchopulmonary dysplasia. Semin Perinatol 2006;30(4):192–9.

90. Miller JD, Carlo WA. Safety and effectiveness of permissive hypercapnia in the preterm infant. Curr Opin Pediatr 2007;19(2):142–4.

91. Kraybill EN, Runyun DK, Bose CL, et al. Risk factors for chronic lung disease in infants with birth weights of 751 to 1000 grams. J Pediatr 1989; 115:115–20.

92. Garland JS, Buck RK, Allred EN, et al. Hypocarbia before surfactant therapy appears to increase bronchopulmonary dysplasia risk in infants with respiratory distress syndrome. Arch Pediatr Adolesc Med 1995;149:617–22.

93. Kamper J, Feilberg Jorgensen N, Jonsbo F, et al. The Danish national study in infants with extremely low gestational age and birthweight (the ETFOL study): respiratory morbidity and outcome. Acta Paediatr 2004;93:225–32.

94. Carlo WA, Stark AR, Wright LL, et al. Minimal ventilation to prevent bronchopulmonary dysplasia in extremely-low-birth-weight infants. J Pediatr 2002; 141:370–4.

95. Woodgate PG, Davies MW. Permissive hypercapnia for the prevention of morbidity and mortality in mechanically ventilated newborn infants. Cochrane Database Syst Rev 2001;(2):CD002061.

96. Thompson WK, Marchak BE, Froese AB, et al. High frequency oscillation compared with standard ventilation in pulmonary injury model. J Appl Phys 1982;52:543–8.

97. Truog WE, Standaert TA, Murphy J, et al. Effect of high frequency oscillation on gas exchange and pulmonary phospholipids in experimental hyaline membrane disease. Am Rev Respir Dis 1983;127: 585–9.

98. Hamilton PP, Onayemi A, Smyth JA, et al. Comparison of conventional and high-frequency ventilation: oxygenation and lung pathology. J Appl Phys 1983;55(1 Pt 1):131–8.

99. Bell RE, Kuehl TJ, Coalson JJ. High-frequency ventilation compared to conventional positive-pressure ventilation in the treatment of hyaline membrane disease. Crit Care Med 1984;12:764.

100. Ackerman NB Jr, Coalson JJ, Kuehl TJ, et al. Pulmonary interstitial emphysema in the premature baboon with hyaline membrane disease. Crit Care Med 1984;12(6):512–6.

101. Boros SJ, Mammel MC, Coleman JM, et al. Comparison of high-frequency oscillatory ventilation and high-frequency jet ventilation in cats with normal lungs. Pediatr Pulmonol 1989;7(1):35–41.

102. DeLemos RA, Coalson JJ, Gerstmann DR, et al. Ventilatory management of infant baboons with hyaline membrane disease: the use of high frequency ventilation. Pediatr Res 1987;21:594–602.

103. Meredith KS, deLemos RA, Coalson JJ, et al. Role of lung injury in the pathogenesis of hyaline membrane disease in premature baboons. J Appl Phys 1989;66(5):2150–8.

104. Cotton CM, Clark RH. High-frequency oscillatory ventilation. In: Spitzer AR, editor. Intensive care of the fetus and neonate. 2nd edition. Philadelphia: Elsevier Mosby; 2005. p. 671–9.

105. Lampland AL, Mammel MC. The role of high-frequency ventilation in neonates: evidence-based recommendations. Clin Perinatol 2007;34:129–44.

106. Vitali SH, Arnold JH. Bench-to-bedside review: ventilator strategies to reduce lung injury – lessons from pediatric and neonatal intensive care. Crit Care 2005;9(2):177–83.

107. Courtney SE, Durand DJ, Asselin JM, et al. High frequency oscillatory ventilation versus conventional mechanical ventilation for very-low-birth weight infants. N Engl J Med 2002;347:643–52.

108. Johnson AH, Peacock JL, Greenough A, et al. High frequency oscillatory ventilation for the prevention of chronic lung disease of prematurity. N Eng J Med 2002;347:633–42.

109. Van Kaam AH, Rimesberger PC. Lung-protective ventilation strategies in neonatology: what do we know–what do we need to know? Crit Care Med 2007;35(3):925–31.

110. Henderson-Smart DJ, Bhuta T, Cools F, et al. Elective high frequency oscillatory ventilation versus conventional ventilation for acute pulmonary dysfunction in preterm infants. Cochrane Database Syst Rev 2003;(4):CD000104.

111. Clark RH, Gerstmann DR, Null DM Jr, et al. Prospective randomized comparison of high-frequency oscillatory and conventional ventilation in respiratory distress syndrome. Pediatrics 1992; 89(1):5–12.

112. Gerstmann DR, Minton SD, Stoddard RA, et al. The Provo multicenter early high-frequency oscillatory ventilation trial: improved pulmonary and clinical outcome in respiratory distress syndrome. Pediatrics 1996;98(6 part 6):1044–57.

113. Henderson-Smart DJ, Cools F, Bhuta T, et al. Elective high frequency oscillatory ventilation versus conventional ventilation for acute pulmonary dysfunction in preterm infants. Cochrane Database Syst Rev 2007;(3):CD000104.

114. Bhuta T, Henderson-Smart DJ. Elective high-frequency oscillatory ventilation versus conventional ventilation in preterm infants with pulmonary dysfunction: systematic review and meta-analyses. Pediatrics 1997;100(5):E6.

115. Joshi VH, Bhuta T. Rescue high frequency jet ventilation versus conventional ventilation for severe pulmonary dysfunction in preterm infants. Cochrane Database Syst Rev 2006;1:CD000437.

116. Keszler M, Modanlou HD, Brudno DS, et al. Multicenter controlled clinical trial of high frequency jet ventilation in preterm infants with uncomplicated respiratory distress syndrome. Pediatrics 1997;4 593–9.

117. Keszler M. High frequency ventilation: evidence based practice and specific clinical indications. NeoReviews 2006;7(5):e234–48.

118. Bernstein G, Mannino FL, Heldt GP, et al. Randomized multicenter trial comparing synchronized and conventional intermittent mandatory ventilation in neonates. J Pediatr 1996;128(4):453–63.

119. Chan V, Greenough A. Randomised controlled trial of weaning by patient triggered ventilation or conventional ventilation. Eur J Pediatr 1993 152:51–4.

20. Chen J-Y, Ling U-P, Chen J-H. Comparison of synchronized and conventional intermittent mandatory ventilation in neonates. Acta Paediatr Jpn 1997;39:578–83.

21. Donn SM, Nicks JJ, Becker MA. Flow-synchronized ventilation of preterm infants with respiratory distress syndrome. J Perinatol 1994;14:90–4.

22. Baumer JH. International randomised controlled trial of patient triggered ventilation in neonatal respiratory distress syndrome. Arch Dis Child Fetal Neonatal Ed 2000;82:F5–10.

23. Beresford MW, Shaw NJ, Manning D. Randomised controlled trial of patient triggered and conventional fast rate ventilation in neonatal respiratory distress syndrome. Arch Dis Child Fetal Neonatal Ed 2000;82:F14–8.

24. Claure N, Bancalari E. New modes of mechanical ventilation in the preterm newborn: evidence of benefit. Arch Dis Child Fetal Neonatal Ed 2007; 92:F508–12.

125. Greenough A, Dimitriou G, Prendergast M, et al. Synchronized mechanical ventilation for respiratory support in newborn infants. Cochrane Database Syst Rev 2008;1:CD000456.

126. Muscedere JG, Mullen JB, Gan K, et al. Tidal ventilation at low airway pressures can augment lung injury. Am J Respir Crit Care Med 1994;149:1327–34.

127. Dreyfuss D, Saumon G. Ventilator-induced lung injury: lessons from experimental studies. Am J Respir Crit Care Med 1998;157:294–323.

128. Naik AS, Kallapur SG, Bachurski CJ, et al. Effects of ventilation with different positive end-expiratory pressures on cytokine expression in the preterm lamb lung. Am J Respir Crit Care Med 2001;164: 494–8.

Approach to Diagnosing Congenital Cardiac Disorders

Georgios A. Hartas, MD, Emmanouil Tsounias, MD, Monesha Gupta-Malhotra, MBBS*

KEYWORDS

- Congenital heart malformations • Cyanosis • Neonate
- Hyperoxia test • Chest x-ray • Electrocardiogram
- Patent ductus arteriosus • Physical examination

The subspecialty of pediatric cardiology has rapidly progressed in the past 60 years, with rapid development of centers for management of congenital heart disease (CHD) all around the world. Major advances have included development of echocardiography, including fetal echocardiography, interventional cardiac catheterization, electrophysiology, and improved cardiopulmonary bypass and surgical techniques. The use of prostaglandins to keep the ductus arteriosus open has greatly contributed in this progress. Congenital cardiac defects affect approximately 0.8% to 3.5% of children.[1] CHD is among the major causes of in utero demise and is a major congenital human malformation. This article reviews the approach to diagnosing CHD in a newborn.

CYANOTIC AND ACYANOTIC CONGENITAL CARDIAC DEFECTS

Congenital heart diseases can be separated into cyanotic and acyanotic defects, or ductal-dependent and ductal-independent lesions.

Cyanotic Cardiac Defects

A decrease in pulmonary blood flow or obstruction in pulmonary blood flow may account for deep cyanosis (**Table 1**). However, there are lesions in which the deoxygenated blood mixes with oxygenated blood, giving rise to mild cyanosis and eventually increased pulmonary blood flow. This mild cyanosis may not be visible to the naked eye in the early phases and may only be detected by a pulse oximetry reading. Lesions with single ventricular physiology may be associated with increased or decreased pulmonary blood flow and can present as a mixing or an obstructed lesion, respectively (see **Table 1**). Neonates with cyanosis do not always have CHD. Cyanosis may result from respiratory disease or central nervous system disorders. When in doubt, the arterial blood gas is confirmatory. In addition, one should determine if the cyanosis is intermittent or constant. Gastroesophageal reflux can cause intermittent cyanosis that is also associated with apnea. D-transposition of the great arteries is the most common cause of central cyanosis in the first month of life; tetralogy of Fallot is the most common cause of cyanosis after the first month of life.

Acyanotic Cardiac Defects

Acyanotic cardiac defects are seldom associated with cyanosis unless there is associated lung pathology or increased pulmonary-vascular resistance (**Table 2**). The shunt lesions, typically an atrial or ventricular septal defect, atrioventricular canal defects or a patent ductus arteriosus (PDA), are usually associated with increasing left-to-right shunting, with falling pulmonary vascular resistance in the first 4 to 6 weeks after birth. If the pulmonary vascular resistance does not decrease, there may be no evidence for shunting or pulmonary congestion, despite a large septal defect. These lesions are also associated with murmurs; however, the murmurs may not be heard

Division of Cardiology, Department of Pediatrics, University of Texas Health Science Center, Children's Memorial Hermann Hospital, Houston, TX, 77030, USA
* Corresponding author.
E-mail address: monesha.gupta@uth.tmc.edu (M. Gupta-Malhotra).

Crit Care Nurs Clin N Am 21 (2009) 27–36
doi:10.1016/j.ccell.2008.10.003

ccnursing.theclinics.com

Table 1
Cyanotic lesions

	Obstructive Lesions (Decreased PBF)	Nonobstructive Lesions (Increased PBF)
Lesions	TOF Tricuspid atresia/VSD/PS PS/IVS Ebstein's anomaly Single ventricle with PS Infracardiac TAPVR	d-TGA/VSD Tricuspid atresia/VSD/no PS Truncus arteriosus Single ventricle without PS Supracardiac or cardiac TAPVR without obstruction
Symptoms	Dusky, FTT, (breathing difficulty with Ebstein's anomaly, TAPVR)	Mild duskiness, FTT, breathing difficulty, diaphoresis
Signs	Cyanosis, usually moderate to severe,[a] hypercyanotic spells, murmur	Mild cyanosis, tachypnea, murmur
CXR	Hypoxemic lungs, usually normal heart size (cardiomegaly with Ebstein's anomaly), RDS picture with TAPVR	Pulmonary vascular congestion (overcirculation), cardiomegaly
EKG	RAH, RVH, RBBB	RVH, BVH
ECHO	To define the anatomy, function and hemodynamics	
Cardiac cath	To evaluate hemodynamics, define intracardiac and extracardiac anatomy, BAS, stent placement, balloon valvuloplasty and angioplasty	

Abbreviations: BAS, Ballon atrial septostomy; BVH, biventricular hypertrophy; CXR, chest roentgenogram; d-TGA, d-Transposition of the great arteries; FTT, failure to thrive; IVS, intact ventricular septum; PBF, pulmonary blood flow; PS, pulmonary stenosis; RAH, right atrial hypertrophy; RBBB, right bundle branch block; RDS, respiratory distress syndrome; RVH, right ventricular hypertrophy; TAPVR, total anomalous pulmonary venous return; TOF, tetralogy of Fallot; VSD, ventricular septal defect.
[a] Cyanosis depends upon the degree of pulmonary obstruction.

early when there is high pulmonary-vascular resistance and a small left-to-right shunt.

Ductal-Independent Lesions

The pulmonary blood flow or the systemic blood flow does not depend on the shunting of the blood via the PDA. Uncomplicated shunt lesions are usually not ductal dependent. Coarctation of aorta can be a progressive lesion that usually develops as

the PDA closes, and may or may not be a ductal-dependent lesion.

Ductal-Dependent Lesions

The ductal-dependent lesions are lesions that require a PDA to be present to shunt blood to the pulmonary artery or to the descending aorta and thus, to the systemic circulation. The lesions that are dependent upon the PDA to provide

Table 2
Acyanotic (shunt) lesions

Lesions	ASD, PAPVR	VSD, PDA
Symptoms[a]	FTT, difficulty breathing, diaphoresis	
Signs	Tachypnea, tachycardia, murmur	Increased SBP and pulse pressure (PDA), tachypnea, tachycardia, murmur
CXR	Increased pulmonary vascular markings, right sided cardiomegaly	Increased pulmonary vascular marking, left sided cardiomegaly (seen better on lateral view)
EKG	RAH, RVH	LAH, LVH, BVH (in large defects)
ECHO	To define anatomy and size of the defect	
Cardiac catheterization	To define anatomy, calculate PVR, calculate Qp:Qs	

Abbreviations: ASD, atrial septal defect; LAH, left atrial hypertrophy; LVH, left ventricular hypertrophy; PAPVR, partial anomalous pulmonary venous return; PDA, patent ductus arteriosus; PVR, pulmonary vascular resistance; Qp, pulmonary blood flow; Qs, systemic blood flow; SBP, systolic blood pressure.
[a] Depends upon size of lesion and pulmonary vascular resistance.

pulmonary blood flow include tricuspid atresia with significant pulmonary stenosis, pulmonary atresia with intact ventricular septum, tetralogy of Fallot with significant pulmonary stenosis or atresia, and Ebstein's anomaly with significant pulmonary stenosis. The lesions that are dependent upon the PDA to provide systemic blood flow include hypoplastic left heart syndrome, critical aortic stenosis, interrupted aortic arch, and significant coarctation of the aorta.

MEDICAL HISTORY

History-taking is the basic step in the cardiac evaluation. It is imperative to establish a good clinical history. The following history-taking is helpful in determining the cause of cyanosis. Many times, an echocardiogram is ordered without the preliminary evaluation, which should be discouraged.

Family History

A history of CHD in close relatives increases the chance of CHD in a neonate. The rate of the CHD in a first-degree relative of a patient with CHD is 1% to 10%; however, this is related to the prevalence of a particular defect.[2–5] For example, bicuspid aortic valve in a parent may be associated with left-heart obstructive lesions in the neonate.[6] Thus, it is important to determine a family history of any cardiac defects, premature sudden death, arrhythmias such as long QT syndrome, and cardiomyopathy.

Obstetric History

A review of the current antenatal course should include history of maternal drugs, medical conditions, substance abuse, and infections. Maternal substance abuse, as for example with alcohol, is associated with fetal alcohol syndrome that can result in septal defects.[7] Maternal use of medications such as phenytoin, an anticonvulsant, can produce heart defects.[8] Maternal lupus erythromatosus has been associated with neonatal congenital heart block.[9] Infants of diabetic mothers have an increased incidence of cardiomyopathy and congenital heart defects.[10] Maternal infections, such as rubella, can result in cardiac anomalies of the fetus, such as PDA.[11] Certain other infections during pregnancy can lead to myocarditis.

Perinatal History

The perinatal history is helpful in determining cyanosis from other etiologies, such as lung disease (meconium aspiration) or central nervous system disease (maternal sedation). Infants with persistent pulmonary hypertension demonstrate right-to-left shunting through a patent foramen ovale or a PDA, and thus mimic a cyanotic heart defect.

Symptoms

Feeding and growth

Poor feeding or tiredness after eating small quantities of food is typical for neonates with shunt lesions. In infants, one should not only determine the volume, but also the feeding duration, as respiratory distress can compromise feeds. Respiratory distress can also further increase the risk of aspiration into the lungs, therefore compromising their function. Growth should be followed closely in all patients with cardiac defects, as lower caloric intake and increased energy needs can result in poor weight gain.

Cyanosis and hypercyanotic spells

Duskiness may or may not be visible to the naked eye. Some lesions with balanced mixing may give rise to mild cyanosis only (see **Table 1**). Other lesions, such as those with severe pulmonary stenosis, may give rise to profound cyanosis (see **Table 1**). Neonates with tetralogy of Fallot or similar physiology, such as a double-outlet right ventricle with pulmonary stenosis or a subaortic ventricular septal defect, may present with hypercyanotic spells with excessive tachypnea and diaphoresis because of sudden spasm of the infundibulum.

Chest pain or excessive crying

Chest pain may be associated with exercise, such as feeding. Lesions with pericarditis, significant left-ventricular outflow obstruction, coronary artery anomaly, such as an anomalous origin of left coronary artery from the pulmonary artery, can give rise to chest pain. In addition, systemic hypertension has been associated with excessive crying in neonates, most likely secondary to headache.

Palpitations, syncope, and pallid spells

The neonate may present with irregular rhythm, bradycardia, or tachycardia. Maternal substance abuse should be determined. Determining the use of cardiac stimulants (nicotine, caffeine) is often helpful in determining the cause of tachycardia. Furthermore, duration, frequency, and associated symptoms are important while taking the history. Occasional premature atrial or ventricular contractions are usually benign findings in the newborn. Supraventricular and ventricular tachycardias, or extreme bradycardias, can be associated with pallor, diaphoresis, dizziness, and syncopal or pallid spells, all related to the decreased cardiac output.

PHYSICAL EXAMINATION

The cardiac examination consists of the following: vital signs, inspection, palpation, and auscultation. The order of the examination should be adjusted to obtain the most information. Usually, auscultation is performed before palpation to minimize irritation of the infant.

Vital Signs

The vital signs, including four extremity blood pressures and oxygen saturations (pre- and post-ductal in infants) should be obtained in every neonate suspected to have heart disease.

Blood pressure

The blood pressure (BP) should be measured in all extremities, preferably the upper arms and the thighs. It is important to measure the BP in both the left and the right arm because of the possibility of an aberrant subclavian artery. The width of the cuff should be of the appropriate size. A falsely elevated BP will be obtained if the cuff is too small. If the systolic BP in the upper extremities is higher than the lower extremities, with more than a 15% difference, then one should consider the diagnosis of a coarctation of the aorta.

Respiratory rate

The respiratory effort and pattern should be observed to distinguish pulmonary disease (grunting, flaring, retracting) from cardiac disease (usually mild tachypnea). Very often, changes in the respiratory rate (tachypnea) and the heart rate (tachycardia) are the first to become abnormal in heart failure, pericardial effusion, pulmonary congestion, or arrhythmias. Obstructed total anomalous pulmonary venous return can present with severe respiratory compromise indistinguishable from severe respiratory distress syndrome.

Heart rate

The normal heart rate of a neonate is 120 to 160 beats per minute. With a heart rate of less than 80 beats per minute (bradycardia), the clinician should investigate the possibility of heart block that can be seen with neonatal lupus, atrioventricular canal defects, or l-transposition of great arteries. Poor cardiac output and poor perfusion can occur with a low heart rate, as the cardiac output in the neonate is often dependent on the heart rate. On the other hand, if the heart rate is more than 180 beats per minute (tachycardia), then one should consider the diagnosis of supraventricular tachycardia that can be associated with Ebstein's anomaly and Wolf-Parkinson-White syndrome. Persistent tachycardia, usually for more than 24 hours, may lead to heart failure.

The metabolic demands of the heart increases, leading to increased caloric expenditure and, thus, failure to thrive with persistent tachycardia. Finally, apnea, seizures, thyroid disorders, and medications such as epinephrine or caffeine can affect the heart rate as well.

Temperature

Hypothermia can lead to desaturation on pulse oximetry because of poor perfusion of the extremities. Medications such as prostaglandin, used in ductal-dependent lesions to maintain patency, may cause hyperthermia. In neonates with central lines, such as umbilical venous or arterial catheters, hyper- or hypothermia should raise the suspicion of endocarditis or thrombophlebitis.

Oxygen saturation via pulse oximetry

Preductal and postductal saturations should be determined. If the preductal saturations are higher than the postductal saurations, one should suspect pulmonary hypertension, with right-to-left shunting at the PDA level (deoxygenated blood from the pulmonary arteries to the descending aorta through the PDA). Other lesions that could cause the previous condition are left ventricular outflow tract obstructions, such as interrupted aortic arch, critical aortic stenosis, and critical coarctation of the aorta. If the postductal saturations are consistently higher than the preductal saturations, then one should suspect d-transposition of the great arteries. In this case, the oxygenated blood will shunt from the pulmonary artery to the descending aorta via the PDA. Certain heart conditions, especially those with single ventricles, should have a lower saturation, ideally between 75% to 85%, to maintain adequate pulmonary and systemic blood flow.

Inspection

General appearance

The general appearance, including size of the neonate (small or large for gestational age) and the presence of dysmorphic features, is important. Certain syndromes, such as Trisomy 13 and Turner syndrome, are associated with high incidence of CHD. Neonates with Down syndrome (Trisomy 21) need to be evaluated for atrioventricular canal defects.[12] Systemic malformations are also associated with CHD. For example, an infant with skeletal abnormalities of upper limbs may have an atrial septal defect (Holt-Oram syndrome).[13] Newborns with CHARGE association (coloboma, heart defect, choanal atresia, growth retardation, genitourinary abnormalities, ear problems) can have associated congenital heart diseases.[14] DiGeorge syndrome is associated with conotruncal heart defects, such as tetralogy of Fallot and double-outlet right ventricle.[15]

Respiratory status

Marked respiratory distress is suggestive of pulmonary pathology or, rarely, pulmonary venous obstruction. A patient with congestive heart failure will present with baseline tachypnea that increases with any effort, such as feeding. Grunting is always pathologic and it often accompanies pulmonary edema.

Color

Central cyanosis is clinically detectable when the arterial saturations are 85% or lower. If the child is anemic, then the cyanosis will be evident with lower saturations. If, on the other hand, the neonate is polycythemic, then the cyanosis will be evident with higher saturations. The cyanosis in CHD is associated with arterial desaturation. The best place to evaluate central cyanosis is the tongue; it has a rich vascular supply and is free of pigmentation. Central cyanosis worsens with crying, feeding, and activity. One should not confuse the above with the peripheral cyanosis or the acrocyanosis. Acrocyanosis is associated with normal saturations and represents a vasomotor phenomenon.

Diaphoresis

Sweating while feeding can be a sign of heart failure. This is because of catecholamine release from the increased sympathetic activity, as a compensatory mechanism for decreased cardiac output.

Palpation

Palpation of the precordium is very important. Up to the first 2 weeks of life, a palpable right ventricular impulse along the left sternal border is considered to be normal. After this period, the finding is considered abnormal. Many forms of CHD are associated with pressure overload (tetralogy of Fallot, d-transposition of the great arteries) or volume overload (large atrial septal defect, atrioventricular canal) of the right ventricle that can cause an increase in the right-ventricular impulse. Displacement of the cardiac impulse outside the nipple line may indicate cardiomegaly.

Peripheral pulses

One should palpate the central pulse simultaneously in the upper and lower extremities. If there is a delay between the upper and the lower extremity pulses, or absence of femoral pulses, then coarctation of the aorta should be considered. If the pulses in all limbs are diminished, this would indicate cardiac failure with low cardiac output or lesion, such as a hypoplastic left heart syndrome. Bounding peripheral pulses reflect aortic run-off lesions, such as a PDA, arteriovenous malformations, or aortic regurgitation.

Edema and signs of fluid overload

Total body-fluid overload can accompany congestive heart failure and, thus, cause peripheral edema and hepatomegaly. Peripheral edema is seen around the eyes, scrotal area, and in the sacral regions in infants because of gravity; this is different from older children who can walk, where the edema is located in the lower extremities, especially in the ankles.

Auscultation

Heart sounds should be evaluated for location (left or right side of chest) and other abnormalities. The first heart sound is heard best at the left lower sternal border or apex of the heart, and the second heart sound at the left upper sternal border. The second heart sound (S2), has two components: the A2 (the aortic valve that closes first) and the P2 (the pulmonic valve that closes thereafter.) In the newborn period and up to approximately 3 weeks of life, when the pulmonary vascular resistance drops to adult levels, the S2 is split and does not vary with the respiration. When the PVR drops to normal, then the S2 is split and varies with the respirations with increased splitting during inspiration. This is a result of the fact that during inspiration, the negative intrathoracic pressure will increase the flow to the right cardiac chambers and thus, more flow will go through the pulmonary valve, delaying its closure. The two components of S2 will be widely split with the above variation, when there will be lesions causing right ventricular volume overload, and also, if right bundle branch block is present. If there are increased pulmonary pressures, then the P2 will be loud, as this will cause the pulmonary valve to close with increased force.

The second heart sound will be single in any defect with only one functioning semilunar valve, such as pulmonary atresia, hypoplastic left heart syndrome, truncus arteriosus, or severe aortic/pulmonary stenosis. The second heart sound will be loud in patients in whom the aorta is relatively close to the sternum, such as d-transposition of great arteries. An S3 gallop is considered normal in the neonatal period, but may occur with enlarged left ventricle; however, an S4 gallop will be indicative of heart failure, usually because of a stiff and noncompliant left ventricle.

Clicks are associated with noise caused by abnormal valves, such as a bicuspid aortic valve. Physiologic murmurs can occur in normal children and are not related to structural abnormalities in

Table 3
Murmurs

	Systolic	Diastolic	Continuous
RUSB	AS, supravalvar AS,	AI	JVH
LUSB	PS, ASD (functional PS), PPS, CoA	PI	PDA, JVH
LLSB	HOCM, VSD, vibratory murmur, TR	TS	Coronary AV fistula, AP collateral
Apex	MR	MS	—

Abbreviations: AS, aortic stenosis; AI, aortic insufficiency; AP, aortopulmonary collateral; AV, arteriovenous; CoA, Coarctation of the aorta; HOCM, hypertrophic obstructive cardiomyopathy; JVH, Jugular venous hum; LUSB, left upper sternal border; LLSB, lower left sternal border; MR, mitral regurgitation; MS, mitral stenosis; PI, pulmonary insufficiency; PPS, peripheral pulmonary stenosis; RUSB, right upper sternal border; TR, tricuspid regurgitation; TS, tricuspid stenosis.

the heart. They are usually soft, systolic, short, and without any signs or symptoms. Abnormal murmurs are associated with disturbed flow across an obstructive lesion, or a shunt lesion (**Table 3**). The location, timing, intensity, and quality of the murmur should be assessed. They are graded from 1 to 6 and murmurs more than grade 4 produce a palpable thrill in the precordium. It is important to realize that the absence of the murmurs will not exclude cardiac defects.

DIAGNOSTIC TESTS
Hyperoxia Test

The hyperoxia test is used to determine whether the cyanosis is cardiac or noncardiac in origin, and can be helpful in the evaluation of the cyanotic neonate. Any infant with saturations obtained via pulse oximetry that are less than 93%, or who has cyanosis, should undergo this test. It consists of obtaining preductal arterial blood-gas measurements and saturations while the child is on room air (FiO_2: 0.21), and then repeating the blood-gas measurements and saturations with the infant on high inspired oxygen (FiO_2: 1.0), for example via an oxy-hood for 10 minutes. If the patient has a cyanotic heart defect, then the PaO_2 will usually be less than 150 mm Hg and the saturations will be less than 85%. If the cyanosis is because of pulmonary and neurologic abnormalities, then PaO_2 will be higher than 150 mm Hg and the saturations will be greater than 85%.[16] Patients with persistent pulmonary hypertension may mimic cyanotic heart disease because of a fixed right to left shunt.

Chest Roentgenogram

A CXR can be helpful to determine the urgency of the patient's condition. The degree of pulmonary vascularity (**Figs. 1** and **2**) and the heart size can also be assessed. An increase in the vascular markings would indicate that the pulmonary blood flow is at least twice the normal amount (see **Fig. 1**)

and may be seen with shunt lesions, such as atrioventricular canal defects and PDA. Decreased pulmonary vascular markings indicate that there is decreased blood flow to the pulmonary arteries (see **Fig. 2**), and can be seen with obstructive lesions, such as tetralogy of Fallot or pulmonary stenosis. The heart is considered enlarged if the cardiothoracic ratio is greater than 0.6 in infants. If there is severe cardiomegaly, one should consider the diagnosis of Ebstein's anomaly.

The shape of the cardiac silhouette may help differentiate between the cardiac defects (**Figs. 3** and **4**). The presence or absence of a thymus should be assessed in a child with DiGeorge syndrome, as the thymus may be absent. Lastly, one should confirm the position of the heart relative to the liver and the stomach bubble, to evaluate for Heterotaxia syndrome (**Fig. 5**).

Electrocardiogram

A 12-lead EKG will assist in determining the rhythm, rate, axis, conduction intervals, atrial and ventricular enlargement, and the ST-T segment

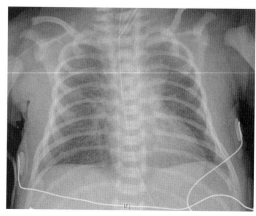

Fig. 1. Increased pulmonary blood flow with prominent perihilar vascular structures in a neonate with complete atrioventricular canal defect.

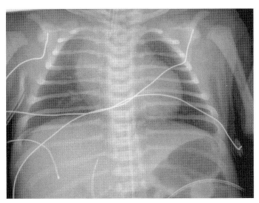

Fig. 2. Cardiomegaly, decreased pulmonary blood flow, and hypoxemic lungs in a neonate with tricuspid atresia.

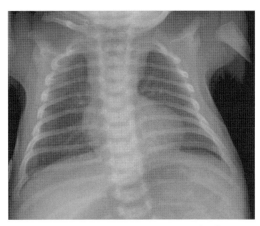

Fig. 4. "Boot shaped heart" in tetralogy of Fallot. Note decreased pulmonary blood flow and hypoxemic lungs.

morphology. In the newborn period, the QRS axis is deviated to the right, indicating predominance of the right ventricular forces, because in utero the right ventricle is the "systemic" ventricle, pumping most of the blood to the pulmonary arteries and via the PDA to the descending aorta. If there is a left-axis deviation, then this will imply an abnormality (**Fig. 6**). The axis will eventually deviate to the left after few months. If an EKG shows left ventricular hypertrophy (see **Fig. 6**), then one should consider heart lesions, such as a PDA, ventricular septal defect, or aortic stenosis. If, on the other hand, the EKG shows right ventricular hypertrophy (**Fig. 7**), then one should consider lesions such as pulmonary stenosis, tetralogy of Fallot, atrial septal defect, and anomalous pulmonary venous return. Rhythm disturbances, Wolf-Parkinson-White syndrome, and long QT syndrome and other conduction defects (**Fig. 8**) can also be determined by an EKG.

Echocardiogram

The echocardiogram is one of the most valuable tools and has revolutionized the field of pediatric cardiology. A transthoracic echocardiogram can provide anatomic diagnosis, as well functional information (**Fig. 9**). Most children with congenital heart defects today go to surgery based on echocardiographic findings, without the need for additional imaging and cardiac catheterization. However, extracardiac structures are better evaluated by another imaging modality, such as magnetic resonance imaging or angiography. Fetal echocardiography is helpful in diagnosing heart defects (**Fig. 10**), determining the size and the function of the heart, and evaluating for rhythm disturbances. Transesophageal echocardiography uses a flexible endoscope with a transducer

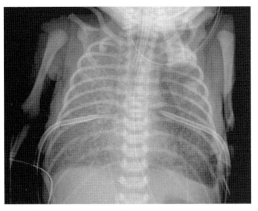

Fig. 3. "Snowman" sign with supracardiac total anomalous pulmonary venous return. Increased interstitial congestion and edema (reticular pattern). Pneumothorax with chest tubes in place.

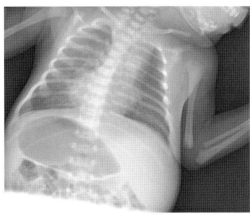

Fig. 5. Chest X-ray. Note abdominal situs inversus with stomach bubble to the right and liver to the left and also note dextrocardia.

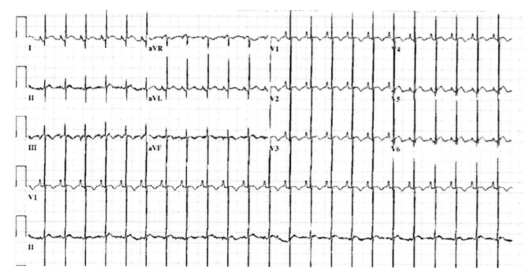

Fig. 6. EKG showing increased voltages in the left precordial leads suggestive of left ventricular hypertrophy. Also note the left superior axis deviation in this patient with atrioventricular canal defect.

at its end, which is inserted in the esophagus to obtain images of the heart while the patient is undergoing heart surgery or in an older patient when the transthoracic echocardiogram pictures are suboptimal. In addition, therapeutic procedures, such as a balloon atrial septostomy, can be performed under echocardiogram guidance. A routine pediatric echocardiogram uses M-mode acquisition, Doppler mapping, and two-dimensional imaging.

M-mode evaluates the dimensions of the cardiac chambers and vessels, and the thickness of the free walls and the ventricular septum. It also calculates the ejection fraction and the shortening fraction. Two-dimensional imaging is used to determine the structure of the heart and demonstrate the spatial relationship of the structures of the heart. The Doppler study helps to detect the direction of the blood flow, the disturbances of the blood flow such as valve regurgitation, the presence of a shunt, and determines pressure gradients. Doppler is also used to estimate the pulmonary artery pressures in the absence of significant shunt lesions and pulmonary stenosis.

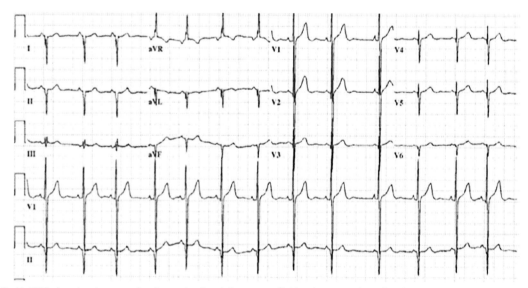

Fig. 7. EKG showing increased voltages in the right precordial leads suggestive of right ventricular hypertrophy. Note upright T-waves in V1 in a 2-week-old infant, suggestive of right ventricular hypertrophy.

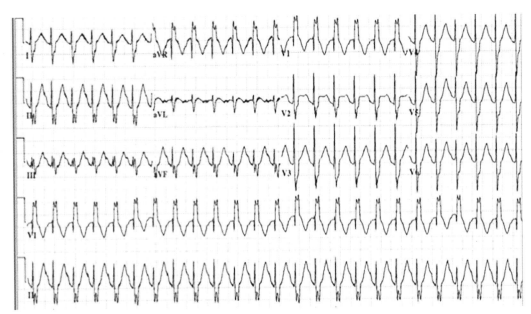

Fig. 8. EKG showing sinus rhythm at 150 beats per minute with right bundle branch block, with widened QRS complexes. Note P-waves before the QRS complexes buried in T-waves, best seen in leads II and III; hence, this is not a ventricular tachycardia.

Cardiac Magnetic Resonance Imaging and Computer Tomography

Cardiac magnetic resonance (CMR) imaging and CT are other techniques applied for cardiac imaging of structures that are not easily seen by echocardiogram, especially those structures covered by the air-filled lungs. CMR in particular is used frequently, as it has no radiation exposure. CMR is extremely useful in delineating the distal branch pulmonary artery anatomy, aortic arch anatomy and postoperative evaluation of baffles, extracardiac conduits, and palliative shunts. CT scan is useful as it requires a shorter imaging time and can image structures containing stents and other devices.

Cardiac Catheterization

Cardiac catheterization and angiography are done using catheters that are placed in the central blood vessels and advanced to the heart under fluoroscopy. The hemodynamic data and the oxygen saturations are recorded from the different cardiac chambers and the major vessels. From the oxygen saturations, one can calculate the magnitude of

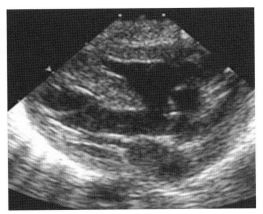

Fig. 9. Transthoracic echocardiogram with a two-dimensional image, showing a ventricular septal defect and an overriding aorta.

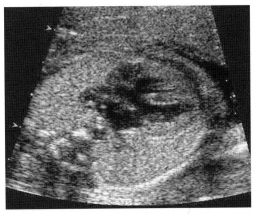

Fig. 10. Fetal echocardiogram with a two-dimensional image showing a ventricular septal defect and an overriding aorta.

the shunting. Finally, selective cineangiography can provide data about the anatomy and function.

Therapeutic procedures, such as a balloon atrial septostomy, can be performed by cardiac catheterization. Catheter-delivered device closure of a PDA or septal defects have eliminated the need for surgical procedures. The special inflatable balloon catheters are now routinely used to relieve obstruction, across vessels and valves, found in critical aortic or pulmonary valvular stenosis, for example.

In summary, an approach to the diagnosis of CHD in a neonate should be a systematic one. The pediatric cardiologist should be called after the preliminary evaluation is completed. It may be difficult to distinguish distress caused by respiratory or cardiac etiologies, and thus, the importance of an organized approach to the physical assessment of the neonate in distress.

REFERENCES

1. Gupta-Malhotra M, Dave A, Sturhan BC, et al. Prevalence of undiagnosed congenital cardiac defects in older children. Cardiol Young 2008;18(4):392–6.
2. Loffredo CA, Chokkalingam A, Sill AM, et al. Prevalence of congenital cardiovascular malformations among relatives of infants with hypoplastic left heart, coarctation of the aorta, and d-transposition of the great arteries. Am J Med Genet A 2004;124A(3):225–30.
3. Maestri NE, Beaty TH, Liang KY, et al. Assessing familial aggregation of congenital cardiovascular malformations in case-control studies. Genet Epidemiol 1988;5(5):343–54.
4. Emanuel R, Withers R, O'Brien K, et al. Congenitally bicuspid aortic valves. Clinicogenetic study of 41 families. Br Heart J 1978;40(12):1402–7.
5. Lewin MB, McBride KL, Pignatelli R, et al. Echocardiographic evaluation of asymptomatic parental and sibling cardiovascular anomalies associated with congenital left ventricular outflow tract lesions. Pediatrics 2004;114(3):691–6.
6. Cripe L, Andelfinger G, Martin LJ, et al. Bicuspid aortic valve is heritable. J Am Coll Cardiol 2004;44(1):138–43.
7. Burd L, Deal E, Rios R, et al. Congenital heart defects and fetal alcohol spectrum disorders. Congenit Heart Dis 2007;2(4):250–5.
8. Lindhout D, Meinardi H, Meijer JW, et al. Antiepileptic drugs and teratogenesis in two consecutive cohorts: changes in prescription policy paralleled by changes in pattern of malformations. Neurology 1992;42(4 Suppl 5):94–110.
9. Friedman DM, Rupel A, Buyon JP. Epidemiology, etiology, detection, and treatment of autoantibody-associated congenital heart block in neonatal lupus. Curr Rheumatol Rep 2007;9(2):101–8.
10. Abu-Sulaiman RM, Subaih B. Congenital heart disease in infants of diabetic mothers: echocardiographic study. Pediatr Cardiol 2004;25(2):137–40.
11. Gittenberger-de Groot AC, Moulaert AJ, Hitchcock JF. Histology of the persistent ductus arteriosus in cases of congenital rubella. Circulation 1980;62(1):183–6.
12. Freeman SB, Bean LH, Allen EG, et al. Ethnicity, sex, and the incidence of congenital heart defects: a report from the National Down Syndrome Project. Genet Med 2008;10(3):173–80.
13. Bossert T, Walther T, Gummert J, et al. Cardiac malformations associated with the Holt-Oram syndrome—report on a family and review of the literature. Thorac Cardiovasc Surg 2002;50(5):312–4.
14. Kallen K, Robert E, Mastroiacovo P, et al. CHARGE association in newborns: a registry-based study. Teratology 1999;60(6):334–43.
15. Oh AK, Workman LA, Wong GB. Clinical correlation of chromosome 22q11.2 fluorescent in situ hybridization analysis and velocardiofacial syndrome. Cleft Palate Craniofac J 2007;44(1):62–6.
16. Sasidharan P. An approach to diagnosis and management of cyanosis and tachypnea in term infants. Pediatr Clin North Am 2004;51(4):999–1021, ix.

Congenital Cardiac Disease in the Newborn Infant: Past, Present, and Future

Sharyl L. Sadowski, MS, APN, NNP-BC

KEYWORDS

- Cardiac • Heart • Newborn • Neonate
- Defects • Management

Congenital heart defects are the most common of all congenital malformations, with a review of the literature reporting the incidence at 6 to 8 per 1000 live births. The Centers for Disease Control[1] reports cyanotic heart defects occurred in 56.9 per 100,000 live births in the United States in 2005, with higher rates noted when maternal age exceeded 40 years. The incidence of congenital heart disease (CHD) in premature infants is 12.5 per 1000 live births, excluding isolated patent ductus arteriosus (PDA) and atrial septal defect (ASD).[2] Despite advances in detection and treatment, CHD accounts for 3% of all infant deaths and 46% of death from congenital malformations.[3]

The past decade has changed the face of congenital cardiac disease in newborn infants. Until the twentieth century, little was known about CHD and, in many cases, the anomaly led to death. Since the early 1990s, survival and quality of life in infants with CHD have improved. There are now an estimated million adults living with complex CHD that required surgery in the neonatal period.[4]

Advances in fetal echocardiography have increased the number of patients diagnosed prenatally, allowing for extensive parental counseling, initiation of prostaglandin therapy in the delivery room, and delivery in a hospital with a pediatric cardiac surgery center.[5,6] In the past 10 years, advances in echocardiography, angiography, interventional catheterization, and more complete knowledge of newborn physiology have improved diagnostic capability while decreasing risk to the patient. Development of the computerized Congenital Heart Surgery Database has allowed clinicians from around the world to compare outcomes of over 40,000 patients.[7] Newer surgical techniques are being developed to allow for total correction of many congenital cardiac defects, while limiting time spent on continuous cardiopulmonary bypass (CPB) or in deep hypothermia with circulatory arrest.[8] Another innovation is miniaturization of CPB systems, reducing circuit priming from 500 mL or more to a range from 140 mL–260 mL, and heparin or poly-2-methoxyethylacrylate coating of circuits before use in neonates.

Today, 96% of newborns with a congenital heart malformation who survive the first year of life will still be alive at 16 years of age.[9] However, this survival is marked with neurodevelopmental morbidities. While overall intelligence is spared, 79% of school-age patients function at age-appropriate levels, 66% have attention deficit hyperactivity disorder, 37% have moderate disabilities, and 6% have severe neurodevelopmental disabilities. These disabilities have been identified as fine and gross motor deficits, visual-motor integration deficits, speech and language impairment, behavioral problems, and low self-esteem.[10] While morbidities have been linked to time spent on CPB or in deep hypothermic circulatory arrest during corrective surgery, recent studies have concluded that many term newborns

Perinatal Center, Division of Obstetrics and Gynecology, University of Illinois at Chicago, 820 South Wood Street, W-210, M/C 808, Chicago, IL 60612, USA
E-mail address: sharyls@uic.edu

Crit Care Nurs Clin N Am 21 (2009) 37–48
doi:10.1016/j.ccell.2008.10.001

ccnursing.theclinics.com

with congenital cardiac defects have white and gray matter brain abnormalities before surgical intervention.[10,11] Brain tissue alterations may be due to changes in cerebrovascular blood flow in the fetus with congenital heart defects, or as a result of the defect itself.[12] The article discusses the embryology, pathogenesis, clinical presentation, incidence, classifications, and management of CHDs.

EMBRYOLOGY AND PATHOGENESIS

The fetal heart begins forming around the 18th day of pregnancy with the formation of a heart tube. This tube elongates and develops dilatations and contractions that form the ventricle and outflow tracts. Abnormal development during this time results in corrected transposition and dextrocardia. The atrial septum and ventricular septum are formed during the fourth and fifth week of fetal life. Abnormal development may result in ventricular septal defect (VSD), ASD, and atrioventricular canal, and absence, stenosis, or atresia of the tricuspid or mitral valves. The single truncus arteriosus separates into the aorta and pulmonary arteries around this time. Abnormal truncal septation may result in truncus arteriosus, tetralogy of Fallot (TOF), pulmonary or aorta valve atresia or stenosis, transposition of the great vessels (TGV), or double-outlet right ventricle. The fetal heart beats with normal sinus rhythm by 16 weeks' gestation.[13]

Fetal circulation differs from postnatal circulation. In utero, the lungs are not needed for gas exchange. Thus the majority of blood from the right ventricle bypasses the lungs going through the ductus arteriosus, which connects the pulmonary artery and aorta. Normal neonatal circulation with blood going to the lungs for gas exchange depends on closure of the ductus arteriosus and foramen ovale soon after birth.

Other factors are associated with cardiac lesions. Male gender is seen more frequently in coarctation of the aorta, aortic stenosis, TGV, and hypoplastic left heart syndrome (HLHS). Female gender is associated with ASD and PDA.[14] Recurrence risk increases by three- to fourfold when a parent or sibling has congenital cardiac disease and increases by 10-fold if two first-order relatives have CHD.[15]

The incidence of CHD is listed above with 90% of the cases due to multifactorial causes, 8% chromosomal/genetic factors, and 2% from environmental teratogens. The most common chromosomal abnormalities associated with a heart defect are Down syndrome; trisomies 13 and 18; Turner syndrome;[16] 22q11 deletion syndromes, including DiGeorge deletion; and Williams, Alagille, and Noonan syndromes. Many teratogens have been identified in the past 20 years, with thalidomide being one of the most well known. Anticonvulsants have been shown to cause coarctation of the aorta, pulmonary stenosis, and PDA.[2] Phenytoin and valproic acid are known to cause coarctation of the aorta, VSD, TGV, TOF, HLHS, pulmonary atresia, aortic stenosis, and pulmonic stenosis. Lithium is associated with Ebstein anomaly, ASD, and tricuspid atresia. Alcohol is known to cause VSD, ASD, coarctation of the aorta, and TOF. A recent study found that use of angiotensin-converting enzyme inhibitor during the first trimester was associated with a 2.9% incidence of a major congenital malformation, including ASD, VSD, and pulmonic stenosis.[17] Other factors include maternal disease states and viral infections. Compared to pregnant women without diabetes, insulin-dependent diabetic women with poor glucose control have five times greater risk of bearing a child with cardiac anomalies, including cardiomyopathy, VSD, double-outlet right ventricle, TGV, truncus arteriosus, and coarctation of the aorta. Recently, maternal obesity has been linked to CHD.[18] Rubella is the only viral illness associated with an increase in congenital cardiac defects, such as PDA, pulmonary stenosis, VSD, and ASD.

CLINICAL PRESENTATION

Cyanosis may be the only evidence of a cardiac lesion in the first week of postnatal life. However, it is not apparent until at least 5 g of hemoglobin per deciliter is desaturated. Thus, cyanosis is influenced by anemia, polycythemia, and 2,3-diphosphoglycerate levels in the newborn. Peripheral or acrocyanosis, which results from sluggish blood flow through the extremities, is normal in the immediate postnatal period and may last several days. Central cyanosis results from desaturated blood exiting the heart and shows itself as a bluish discoloration of the tongue and mucous membranes.

Tachypnea (respiratory rate >60 breaths/min) without dyspnea is an important sign. It is significant if the newborn also has difficulty feeding and must stop feeding to catch its breath. This is a hallmark sign of congestive heart failure (CHF). Hyperpnea may be present in congenital heart lesions that result in decreased pulmonary blood flow. Crying causes increase in oxygen consumption and may exacerbate cyanosis.

Heart sounds may be affected by the presence of a congenital cardiac defect with a loud S_1 heard with PDA, VSD, total anomalous pulmonary venous return (TAPVR), and TOF. A decreased S_1 may be heard in CHF and myocarditis. Abnormal widening of the S_2 is often heard with ASD, TAPVR, TOF, pulmonary stenosis, and Ebstein anomaly. Murmurs may or may not be auscultated in the newborn period. Systolic ejection murmurs are noted in aortic or pulmonic stenosis, TOF, ASD, and TAPVR. Diastolic murmurs usually indicate a cardiac disorder. Early diastolic murmurs are heard with aortic and pulmonic insufficiency, middiastolic murmurs are heard with increased blood flow across the mitral and tricuspid valves, and late-diastolic murmurs are heard with mitral and tricuspid valve stenosis.

Pulses may be affected by certain cardiac defects. Weak pulses are often heard in defects causing left heart outflow obstruction; bounding pulses are associated with PDA, aortic insufficiency, and left-to-right shunts. Blood pressure values depend on gestational age and birth weight.[19] In a healthy full-term infant, average systolic pressure is normally 56–77 mm Hg, average diastolic pressure is normally 33–50 mm Hg, and mean arterial pressure is normally 42–60 mm Hg.[20] Comparison of upper- and lower-extremity pressures should be done. Coarctation of the aorta and aortic arch abnormalities are suggested when systolic blood pressure in the upper extremities is 20 mm Hg greater than that of the lower extremities. Ideally, four-extremity pressures should be obtained. Neonatal hypertension in a term infant is systolic blood pressure greater than 90 mm Hg and a diastolic pressure greater than 60 mm Hg. In a preterm infant, the values are systolic pressure greater than 80 mm Hg and diastolic pressure greater than 50 mm Hg.

CHF may present at different times postnatally. If present at birth, CHF may indicate HLHS, severe tricuspid or pulmonary regurgitation, or fetal supraventricular tachycardia. In the first week of life, CHF is associated with TGV, PDA, or TAPVR. CHF presenting at 1 to 4 weeks of life may indicate critical aortic or pulmonary stenosis or coarctation of the aorta.[15] The hallmark sign of CHF that presents in the neonatal period is poor perfusion which results in, pale, cyanotic, or gray coloring, poor capillary refill, and diaphoresis. Examination reveals tachypnea, tachycardia, active precordium, and hepatomegaly.[21]

Diagnostic studies include arterial blood gas, hyperoxia test, pulse oximetry, chest radiograph, ECG, echocardiography, MRI, and cardiac catheterization. See the article by Hartas and colleagues elsewhere in this issue for a detailed review of these diagnostic modalities.

DEFECT CLASSIFICATION

Congenital cardiac defects are classified using different systems. They can be divided into cyanotic and acyanotic lesions. Cyanotic defects include HLHS, aortic stenosis, coarctation of the aorta, interrupted aortic arch, TOF, TGV, tricuspid atresia, truncus arteriosus, hypoplastic right heart syndrome, Ebstein's anomaly, and aortic stenosis.[22] Acyanotic defects include VSD, ASD, and PDA. Another way of classifying the lesions uses pulmonary blood flow, which is either increased or decreased. Defects with increased pulmonary blood flow include PDA, VSD, ASD, atrioventricular canal, coarctation of the aorta, and aortic stenosis.[22,23] Cardiac lesions with decreased pulmonary blood flow are TOF, pulmonary stenosis, pulmonary atresia, and tricuspid atresia. The third classification system sorts defects according to patency of the ductus arteriosus. Ductal-dependent lesions depend on continued patency of the ductus arteriosus to supply systemic blood flow. These defects include HLHS, coarctation of the aorta, interrupted aortic arch, critical aortic stenosis, pulmonary stenosis, pulmonary atresia with intact ventricular septum, tricuspid atresia, and TGV.

NON–DUCTAL-DEPENDENT DEFECTS

PDA is the fourth most common lesion and occurs when the ductus arteriosus fails to close within a few days after birth. It is seen in 45% of infants weighing less than 1750 g at birth and 80% of those weighing less than 1200 g at birth.[22] PDA is three times more common in females than males. Neonates with PDA present with increased needs for oxygen and ventilatory support at 4 to 7 days of life. A continuous murmur at the upper left sternal border is heard in 80% to 90% of these patients. The diagnosis is confirmed using echocardiography, which details the size of the defect and documents the direction and volume of blood being shunted through the ductus. Medical management is typically the first step and consists of fluid restriction, diuretics, indomethacin, or ibuprofen.[24] Surgical management is reserved for those infants that fail medical management. The long-term prognosis is excellent.

VSD, the most common congenital heart defect, is found in 1 of every 3000 live births and is characterized by an opening in the septum between the right and left ventricle. Clinical symptoms depend on the size of defect, with small

VSDs being asymptomatic, often accompanied by a high-pitched pansystolic murmur at the left sternal border at 4 to 10 days of life, and 50% to 75% of these close spontaneously. A moderate VSD may present with fatigue at feeding and recurrent respiratory infections. Large VSDs usually present with CHF at 1 to 2 months postnatally. Clinical signs of a large VSD are hepatomegaly; increased precordial activity; and loud, blowing pansystolic murmur at left lower sterna border. The diagnosis is made with echocardiography. Twenty percent of large defects become smaller or close without intervention. Medical management includes digoxin and diuretics. Surgical management can be palliative by using banding of the pulmonary artery to decrease pulmonary blood flow; or corrective surgery can suture or patch the defect through a ventriculotomy. Transcatheter devices may be used on some lesions.[25] Newer approaches are combining surgery and intraoperative device placement in complex muscular VSDs.[7] The mortality rate for VSD is approximately 5% in neonates.

ASD occurs in 1 of every 5000 live births, accounting for 7% to 10% of all cardiac defects, with females twice as likely as males to be affected. An ASD is an abnormal opening in the septum between the left and right atria. If isolated, ASD is usually asymptomatic and unrecognized at birth. Within the first year of life, 50% of infants become symptomatic, presenting with CHF, failure to thrive, recurrent respiratory infections, and systolic murmur at the second intercostal space at the left sternal border. Spontaneous closure may occur in small defects. Medical management of CHF and delayed surgical repair is used to treat ASDs with CHF. Early surgical repair with suturing or patching may be used in patients with intractable CHF. Postsurgical complications include residual shunting, arrhythmias, and embolization of the device.[26] Transcatheter closure devices are used with small ASDs, with the patient needing to weigh a minimum of 8 kg. A recent case report documents successful use of a transcatheter device in a 2.3-kg preterm infant.[27] Implantation of the device is guided by transesophageal echocardiography. Survival is 97% at 5 years and 90% at 10 years after repair.[28]

Atrioventricular canal is seen in 1 of every 9000 live births and is the most common cardiac defect associated with Down syndrome. The defect can range from a simple cleft of the mitral or tricuspid valves to the absence of the entire upper and lower septum. These defects allow left-to-right shunting to occur across the accompanying ASD and VSD with symptoms presenting at 1 to 2 weeks if atrioventricular regurgitation is severe. A clinical examination usually reveals a loud pansystolic murmur at the lower left sternal border, which radiates to the back. Management is aimed at avoiding pulmonary vascular obstructive disease. Medical management consists of digoxin and diuretics to control CHF. Surgical management is primary repair with closure of the ASD and VSD and reconstruction of the mitral and tricuspid valves.[7] Surgery generally takes place before 6 months' postnatal age if complete atrioventricular canal is present and at 6 to 12 months for partial atrioventricular canal.

Truncus arteriosus occurs in 1 of every 33,000 live births, accounting for 1% to 2% of congenital cardiac defects. There are three types: (1) type I, the most common, with a short pulmonary artery coming off the base of the common trunk, which then divides into the right and left arteries; (2) type II, with the right and left pulmonary arteries coming from the posterior surface of the common trunk; and (3) type III, where the right and left pulmonary arteries have separate origins in the lateral walls of the common trunk.[29] Truncus arteriosus presents with CHF, bounding pulses, and widened pulse pressure. Intermittent cyanosis may be seen. A harsh systolic murmur at mid- to lower left sterna border may be heard along with a systolic ejection click with a single S_2 heart sound. Echocardiography is the standard diagnostic adjunct. Medical management is aimed at treating CHF with use of diuretics, digoxin, and angiotensin-converting enzyme inhibitors. Surgical repair is done at 6 to 8 weeks and consists of a homograph between the right ventricle and pulmonary artery, VSD closure using a patch, and separation of the pulmonary arteries from the truncus.[30] Postsurgical mortality is less than 10% and 10- to 20-year survival is more than 80%.

TAPVR occurs in 1 of every 17,000 live births and is characterized by pulmonary veins that drain directly or indirectly into the right atrium. Survival depends on the presence of a patent foramen ovale or ASD. The three types of TAPVR include (1) supracardiac, the most common form, which occurs when the pulmonary veins attach above the diaphragm usually to the superior vena cava; (2) cardiac, which is diagnosed when the pulmonary veins attach directly to the coronary sinus, draining into the right atrium; and (3) infracardiac, the most severe form, which is noted when the pulmonary veins attach below the diaphragm into the portal venous system and drain into the inferior vena cava. TAPVR shunts oxygenated blood directly into the right atrium. As the pulmonary vascular resistance decreases, pulmonary blood flow increases, increasing the flow of blood into the right side of the heart. Clinical manifestations in nonobstructed TAPVR are mild cyanosis, CHF, systolic murmur at the upper left sternal border, and a diastolic rumble at the lower left sternal border. Right ventricular dilatation is present on echocardiography.[31] If an obstruction to the pulmonary venous return is present, the patient will develop pulmonary edema, with symptoms that include profound cyanosis and respiratory distress. Medical management is a temporary measure to relieve signs of CHF and cyanosis. Surgery is aimed at correcting the ASD and transplanting the anomalous veins to the left atrium. The mortality rate for infants who have surgery is 12% to 20%.[32]

DUCTAL-DEPENDENT DEFECTS

Coarctation of the aorta occurs in 3% to 5% of all congenital heart defects[23] and is one the most difficult to diagnose in the fetal period.[33] It is the most common heart defect presenting in the second week of life. It is seen in males more often than females with a 2:1 ratio. Coarctation of the aorta is caused by an area of narrowing at the junction of the transverse aortic arch or the ductus arteriosus. The most common site of constriction is just below the origin of the left subclavian artery. Coarctation before the ductus arteriosus is associated with aortic arch hypoplasia and such other defects as VSD, PDA, and TGV. Clinical symptoms include CHF, which, if severe, results in cardiovascular collapse as the ductus is closing, and, in the lower extremities, mottled, pale, and cool skin and decreased or absent pulses. Higher blood pressure (>15 mm Hg) in the upper extremities is a consistent factor in critical constrictions. Examination reveals different findings based on location of the defect. Murmurs are absent if the defect is postductal, and harsh pansystolic murmurs are heard at the left lower sterna border in preductal lesions. A systolic thrill may be felt at the suprasternal notch. Echocardiography may detect the defect if the ductus arteriosus is patent.[34] MRI may be used to determine the site of the coarctation.[35] Cardiac

catheterization is diagnostic and is usually performed before surgery.

If the baby presents after closure of the ductus arteriosus, medical management is aimed at aggressive management of CHF and prostaglandin E_1 (PGE_1) should be started (**Table 1**). If the neonate is critically ill, palliative balloon angioplasty may be performed and then followed by surgical correction. Surgical correction can be done with resection and end-to-end anastomosis or a subclavian flap repair. One of the major drawbacks of the subclavian patch is loss of pulses in the left arm after surgery, although the pulses are usually restored via collateral circulation. Resection with end-to-end anastomosis is the most common procedure and has a low recoarctation rate of 3%.[36] Surgical mortality remains at 2% to 10%, with hypertension the most common complication.

Aortic stenosis occurs in 1 of every 24,000 live births and is four times more likely in male infants. Stenosis may be subvalvular, valvular, or supravalvular and the left ventricular myocardium is hypertrophied. Valvular stenosis is the most common form and is usually associated with a bicuspid aortic valve. If severe aortic stenosis is present in the fetus, it usually results in hypoplasia of the left ventricle. This condition is usually asymptomatic at birth, with examination revealing a grade II to IV harsh systolic murmur at the right upper sternal border, which radiates to the neck and left lower sterna border, and a thrill at the suprasternal notch. If the defect is severe, CHF will be absent at birth but progresses rapidly as the ductus arteriosus closes, leading to sudden deterioration in the neonate. CHF and shock should be treated aggressively with fluid restriction, digoxin, diuretics, correction of acidosis, antibiotic prophylaxis, and infusion of PGE_1 to prevent hypoxia. Early treatment is preferred with balloon valvuloplasty, which carries a mortality of 11%. Multiple procedures may be needed in childhood.[23,32] One study looked at growth and function of the left heart following balloon

Table 1
Guidelines for administration of prostaglandin E_1 for aggressive management of congestive heart failure

Amount of dextrose 5% in water, dextrose 10% in water or 0.9 normal saline to be added to 500 μg of PGE_1	Resulting concentration PGE_1 μg/mL	Rate mL/kg/h to infuse 0.1 μg/kg/min
250 mL	2	3.0
100 mL	5	1.2
50 mL	10	0.6
25 mL	20	0.3

Data from Taketomo CK, Hodding JH, Kraus DM. Pediatric dosage handbook, 14th edition. Hudson (OH): Lexi-Comp; 2007. p. 82.

valvuloplasty and reported rapid normalization of the size of the left ventricle, with reinterventions common in the first year for residual or recurrent aortic stenosis or iatrogenic aortic regurgitation. However, aortic valve replacement is rarely needed.[37] Surgical management includes aortic valvulotomy or valve replacement and is reserved for those that fail balloon valvuloplasty.[38] Factors increasing mortality for aortic valve replacement include age less than 6 months and lower weight.[39]

TOF, which has an incidence of 1 of every 5000 live births, is the most common cyanotic heart defect. This cardiac defect is comprised of four cardiac anomalies: pulmonary stenosis or absent pulmonary valve, VSD, aorta overriding VSD, and right ventricular hypertrophy. Clinical manifestations depend primarily on restriction of pulmonary blood flow. With severe pulmonary stenosis, blood is shunted right to left through the VSD, resulting in hypoxia and cyanosis. In cases of mild stenosis, shunting is left to right, resulting in CHF. In moderate stenosis, shunting across the VSD is minimal until something causes an imbalance in pulmonary or systemic vascular resistance. Infants with TOF are pink at rest and turn blue when crying, as the crying causes right-to-left shunting. This phenomenon–paroxysmal dyspnea and severe cyanosis–is called a "tet spell" and is common in infants and children with TOF.

Clinical examination of the neonate with severe stenosis reveals marked cyanosis, hypoxia, dyspnea, and harsh grade II to IV systolic murmur with thrill at mid- to upper left sterna border. Chest radiography shows a normal-sized boot-shaped heart with decreased pulmonary vascular markings. Treatment consists of propanolol in hypercyanotic infants, and PGE$_1$ infusion to maintain patency of the ductus arteriosus until surgical management. Corrective surgery is preferred before 6 months of age and includes VSD patch repair and, if necessary, a patch to enlarge the pulmonary outflow tract.[32] If severe stenosis or atresia is present, a palliative Blalock-Taussig shunt is performed with complete repair at a later time.[40] Some centers are now reporting good results using primary repair for neonates with TOF and absent pulmonary valve.[41] Postoperative mortality remains less than 5% for uncomplicated cases, increasing with more severe forms.[7] A recent study reviewed long-term outcomes of patients with TOF, finding that children with TOF had lower intelligence and higher numbers of motor deficits, language disabilities, and attention deficit disorders.[42]

TGV occurs in 1 of every 5000 live births with males affected more than females at a 2:1 ratio. TGV is the most common cardiac cause of cyanosis. In this defect, the pulmonary artery is attached to the left ventricle and the aorta comes off the right ventricle. If no other defect is present, circulation will be parallel. Oxygenated blood from the lung enters the left atrium and ventricle and is recirculated to the lungs via the pulmonary artery. Unoxygenated blood returns to the right atrium and ventricle and returns to the body via the aorta. Mixing occurs at the ductus arteriosus and is required for survival. The neonate presents within 24 hours of birth with cyanosis, which worsens rapidly. Murmurs are uncommon and, if heard, are usually associated with a VSD. Chest radiography may show a cardiac silhouette that is normal in size but with an "egg on a string" appearance. Standard diagnosis is by echocardiography.

Medical management is aimed at alleviating metabolic acidosis and infusing PGE$_1$ to maintain ductal patency until a palliative procedure can be performed.[43] The procedure of choice is a catheter-introduced balloon atrial septostomy to create an ASD. Pulmonary artery banding is another procedure and is used to decrease CHF and prevent pulmonary vascular disease. Surgical management of choice is the arterial switch (Jatene procedure), performed at 1 to 2 weeks of life, which detaches the aorta, coronary arteries, and pulmonary artery and reattaches them to the correct ventricles. This allows for anatomic and physiologic correction. Survival after arterial switch is greater than 98% at 4 years. Reported long-term neurodevelopmental morbidities include fine and gross motor deficits, sensory dysfunction, and speech and language deficits.[44]

HLHS, seen in 2.6 of every 10,000 live births, is responsible for 1% to 4% of all congenital cardiac defects and accounts for 25% of all cardiac deaths in the first week of life.[45] HLHS is characterized by mitral valve stenosis or atresia, hypoplastic left ventricle, aortic valve stenosis or atresia, and hypoplastic aortic arch, which result in an inability of the left heart structures to support systemic circulation. Prior to the early 1980s, all of the patients died, usually in the first week of life. The first successful stage 1 operation was performed in 1980 by Norwood. The Norwood procedure is now the most common palliative procedure in HLHS. Along with the Norwood procedure came PGE$_1$ to maintain ductal patency to provide systemic circulation until surgery is possible. While asymptomatic at birth, clinical status rapidly declines as the ductus arteriosus closes. Signs are tachypnea and dyspnea, CHF at 24 to 48 hours of life, severe mottling, gray pallor, markedly diminished pulses, cardiovascular collapse, and shock. This condition is usually recognized on routine screening obstetric ultrasound with prenatal diagnosis by fetal echocardiography at 18 to 22 weeks. Recent advances in fetal diagnosis have led to interventions in the fetus in an attempt to prevent development of HLHS.[46,47] Postnatal diagnosis is by echocardiography and is used to determine atrioventricular valve function, size of the ascending aorta, and interatrial communication.[48] Echocardiography studies should include Doppler and color-flow mapping.[49]

Until recently, parents were offered three treatment options: comfort care, multistage surgical approach, or cardiac transplantation. Since the late 1990s, survival after either the multistaged surgeries or cardiac transplantation has improved dramatically, leading many clinicians to delete comfort care from their discussions with parents. Initial management includes PGE_1 infusion to maintain or reopen the ductus arteriosus and systemic circulation, inhaled oxygen and nitrogen mixture to provide inspired oxygen of less than 21% to maintain 70% to 85% oxygen saturation. This may maximize systemic blood flow and oxygen saturation.[50] Transcatheter balloon atrial septostomy or transcatheter atrial needle puncture followed by serial balloon dilatations may be done to decompress the left atrium.[51]

The staged Norwood surgical procedure carries an overall mortality of 25% to 40%. The first stage includes division of the pulmonary artery and ligation of the ductus arteriosus, placement of a Gore-Tex shunt to maintain pulmonary blood flow, atrial septectomy to allow for continued pulmonary venous return to the right atrium, and right pulmonary artery connection to the aorta. This stage can be performed on small infants with birth weight greater than 1500 g. Mortality ranges from 10% to 39%. Two newer approaches to this stage include the Sano modification using a right ventricle–to–pulmonary artery conduit, and a hybrid approach involving atrial placement of a stent in the ductus arteriosus along with placement of a pulmonary artery band. The Sano procedure uses a 4- to 6-mm conduit to join the right ventricle and pulmonary artery. Potential advantages of this include improved coronary and end-organ perfusion. Disadvantages are increased volume load on the right ventricle, inadequate pulmonary artery growth, and shunt stenosis or thrombosis.[52] One study reports that aspirin appears to lower the risk of shunt thrombosis and risk of death.[53] The hybrid procedure is performed in a special catheterization suite with cardiac surgical capability.[54] The main advantage of this procedure is that it does not require CPB or deep hypothermic cardiac arrest. Complications include narrowing of the ductus arteriosus, with outcomes similar to those associated with the Norwood procedure.

The second stage, which is done before 6 months of age, is a bidirectional Glenn procedure with anastomosis of the right pulmonary artery to the superior vena cava. Mortality for this stage is less than 9.5%. The third stage, performed at 12–24 months of age, is a modified Fontan procedure, which connects the inferior vena cava to the pulmonary artery and closes the ASD. It carries a mortality risk of 10%. Disadvantages of the multistaged surgical approach include (1) the necessity of two to three open surgeries within 2 years of life and (2) the use of a single ventricle to supply systemic circulation.

Cardiac transplantation is offered at several centers in the United States. The advantage is provision of a structurally and physiologically normal heart in one surgical procedure. However, 25% to 40% of babies die awaiting a donor heart. Of those who receive a transplant, survival rates at 1 year are 79% to 89%. Recent advances in ABO-incompatible heart transplants and use of ventricular-assist devices have increased survival rates. ABO-incompatible heart transplants can be performed in the first months of life because anti-A and anti-B antibodies are usually absent.[55]

Perhaps in no other cardiac defect is there quite the controversy that surrounds treatment of HLHS. Variability in practice differs from region to region, center to center, and practitioner to practitioner in regards to parental discussions, treatment options, and method of cardiopulmonary support during surgery. A recent survey has raised questions on the extreme variability in current practices and suggests the shift from single-center experiences to multicenter and multidisciplinary collaboration.[56]

LONG-TERM OUTCOMES

There are over a million adults alive today who had surgery in the first month of life for complex CHD. This is a result of advancements in diagnostic, therapeutic, surgical, and extracorporeal techniques and improvements in neonatal intensive care medicine. Mortality has decreased dramatically. However, morbidity is well documented. The most concerning of the noted morbidities is that of neurodevelopmental deficits, which are often seen by age 1 year. Adverse outcomes in infancy are, but not limited to, feeding issues in 50% and delays in rolling over, crawling, and walking. Preschool children experience speech and language delays, gross motor deficits presenting as clumsiness, and fine motor deficits affecting drawing and handwriting. Issues in school-age patients are attention deficit hyperactivity disorder, problems with visual-motor integration, and executive planning deficits that lead to difficulty in performing instructions with multiple steps.[57] One study reported the deficits being linked to preoperative brain injury, CPB for surgical procedures, limited interaction with the environment in children with cyanotic CHD, and inconsistent environment during prolonged hospitalizations. The study also reported that the deficits are frequently seen in children with complex cardiac defects.[58]

Factors associated with neurodevelopmental outcomes are gestational age, genetics, type of cardiac defect, seizures within 48 hours of surgery, degree of acidosis, age at time of repair, socioeconomic class, hypoxemia, hypoglycemia, low cardiac output, cardiac arrest, length of hospital stay, ventilator days degree of CHF, and need for and type of circulatory support during surgery.[4] Deep hypothermic cardiac arrest is associated with a period of cerebral ischemia followed by reperfusion, during which central nervous system injury takes place. Continuous CPB exposes the brain to foreign substances, creating an inflammatory response. Other studies have looked at surgical approaches for the initial stage in HLHS and have determined that there is no difference between the approaches, although increased length of stay is related to worse outcomes. Seizures, cerebral palsy, attention deficit hyperactivity disorder, and low IQ scores have been reported in children born with HLHS and rates were consistent with multistaged repair and cardiac transplantation.[59] Despite improvements in surgical methods, central nervous system injury remains at 1% to 5% for infants who have surgery for a cardiac defect.[60]

NURSING IMPLICATIONS

Nursing diagnoses may include ineffective breathing pattern, impaired gas exchange, ineffective airway clearance, altered nutrition (less than body requirements), pain, risk for infection, and delayed growth and development.[61] With each of the ductal-dependent lesions described above, treatment was aimed at preventing or treating CHF. Common signs of CHF in the neonate include tachypnea at rest, tachycardia, arrhythmias, hepatomegaly, rales, and fatigue with feeding. Other signs might include diaphoresis, gallop rhythm, or mottling of the extremities. Treatment goals are to decrease oxygen consumption, provide supplemental oxygen as needed, and correct acidosis, electrolyte disturbances, and hypoglycemia. Fluid restriction is common. Medications include digoxin therapy, diuretics, and inotropic agents. Nesiritide is a newer agent showing promise in patients over 1 month of age with low cardiac output and CHF not responsive to traditional management.[59]

Transporting the neonate with a ductal-dependent cardiac lesion may be difficult. In the past, all neonates placed on PGE_1 requiring transport to another medical facility were intubated and mechanically ventilated before transport. This was done to prevent apnea that may accompany high-dose PGE_1. Recent studies have suggested it may not be necessary to intubate and ventilate these neonates, especially if low-dose PGE_1 is used. However, more studies are needed before a blanket recommendation can be made.[62]

Postoperative nursing includes monitoring (with continuous ECG for tachycardia, bradycardia, fibrillation, and asystole) blood pressure of upper and lower extremities; pulse oximetry for decreasing oxygen saturation; and urinary output with 1 to 2 mL/kg/h being a good indicator of renal perfusion. However, oliguria may be present for 48 hours following CPB. Invasive monitoring is used for arterial pressure. Pronounced variations during mechanical ventilation indicate hypovolemia or early heart failure. Increasing right heart pressures indicate poor ventricular function, tricuspid regurgitation, right ventricular overload, residual shunting, or cardiac tamponade. Pulmonary artery pressure catheters are used when postoperative pulmonary hypertension is expected, as in TAPVR, mitral stenosis, and endocardial cushion repair. Mixed venous oxygen saturation can be obtained from newer pulmonary artery catheters. Left-sided cardiac pressures are monitored using a left atrial line, which is helpful in evaluating systemic ventricular function and pulmonary shunting in patients with mitral valve dysfunction, but poses a high risk of air or particulate embolization.[30]

Hemodynamic management is crucial given that neonates are prone to wide swings in physiologic response, including heart rate, temperature, glucose metabolism, and systemic and pulmonary vascular resistance. Heart failure is the most common postoperative event and may be caused by CPB with peak effect 6 to 18 hours after surgery, arrhythmias, hypovolemia, and left ventricular dysfunction. Heart failure may also result from increased afterload, poor contractility, inadequate systemic venous return, and increased pulmonary vascular resistance. Heart failure is usually made evident by low cardiac output. For babies with heart failure, cardiac output is especially low for babies at a postnatal age of less than 1 month, for babies weighing less than 2.5 kg, and for babies with certain types of defects. Signs are lethargy, gray skin, decreased pedal pulses, capillary refill time of more than 3 seconds, edema, oliguria, low blood pressure, and metabolic acidosis. Treatment includes blood for volume replacement to keep hemoglobin above 12 g/dL for noncyanotic defects and above 15 g/dL for cyanotic lesions; strict intake/output; correction of metabolic disorders; use of pulmonary vasodilating medications PGE_1, nitroglycerin, nitroprusside, and inhaled nitric oxide; sedation; and analgesia.[63] Other pharmaceutical agents to consider are isoproterenol, milrinone, nesiritide, dopamine, or dobutamine,[64] and hydrocortisone for hypotension.[65]

Assessment and treatment of any coagulopathies is essential and may include fresh whole blood to maintain hematocrit of 40% to 45%, cryoprecipitate to aid clotting, platelets, and desmopressin to increase von Willebrand factor. Pulmonary hypertension is another complication seen postoperatively and is increased by hypoxia and acidosis. Hypoglycemia, hypokalemia, and hypocalcemia result in decreased myocardial function. Continuous subcutaneous blood glucose monitoring is reported to be safe and perhaps useful in the postoperative care of the neonate with a cardiac defect, but further research is needed before a recommendation for use can be made.[66]

Pain assessment remains a major challenge in newborn infants, specifically those in critical condition, because they lack adequate compensatory mechanisms. Assessment should use a validated pain scoring scale such as the Premature Infant Pain Profile or the Neonatal Infant Pain Scale. In addition, neonates recovering from cardiac surgery are very sensitive to stressful procedures and interventions, and thus require analgesics and sedatives. These might include intermittent muscular blockade, fentanyl drip, spinal anesthesia blockade combined with general anesthesia, and environmental measures to decrease stimuli.[57]

Developmental care for the postsurgical neonate is encouraged through decreases in noise and lighting, clustering of hands-on care, nonnutritive sucking, use of positional devices and facilitated tucking, and involvement of the family.[67]

PARENTAL SUPPORT

The diagnosis of a congenital cardiac defect is stressful for parents and family members whether made pre- or postnatally. With a diagnosis of CHD, the dream of a normal newborn is shattered and the parents grieve the loss while being challenged to accept the sick newborn. The psychological impact of prenatal diagnosis has not been studied in depth, but recent studies report that prenatal diagnosis did not lessen the stress parents experience after birth.[68] Four factors have been identified that influence reactions at time of diagnosis: approach

used by medical personnel, complexity of the explanation, details of infant's condition, the amount of opportunity to ask questions. Families have stated they prefer to be told about their baby's diagnosis in a private place when another family member could be present. The article by Upham and Medoff-Cooper[69] uses the acronym PACE, which stands for *planning* the setting, *assessing* the family's background knowledge, *choosing* strategies that fit with the individual family's situation, and *evaluating* the family's level of understanding of the information presented. Family-centered care may facilitate families being given accurate education, support, and skills to care for their sick newborn.[70]

Hope, fear, sadness, and anger are normal responses to this diagnosis. Responses to the diagnosis may vary between parents, with fathers feeling a need to be strong and hide their emotions. Parental stress may be increased when there are siblings needing care at home, one or both parents needing to be at work, and pressing financial concerns. The influence of prior experiences and of values, culture, and religion may also affect stress. Support options for parents may include parental support groups, clergy, social workers, or formal counseling. Following surgery, one of the most stressful times for parents of infants with CHD may be at discharge. Stress may be reduced through written or audio- and video-taped parent education materials that are accurate and easily understood, and by encouraging parents to participate in their infant's care while in the ICU and during hospital stay, a safe environment for the parents to gain confidence in preparation for caring for their baby at home.[69]

SUMMARY

Most neonates are born healthy. However, 6 to 8 of every 1000 live birth results in a newborn infant with CHD with this rate increasing with advanced maternal age and prematurity. Until the twentieth century, the majority of these newborns died because treatment was not available. With the advances made in the field of fetal and pediatric cardiology, survival and quality of life have improved, especially in the past 10–20 years. Significant advancements have been made in fetal echocardiography, leading to earlier prenatal parental discussions and treatment decisions; in postnatal echocardiography and angiography, leading to greater accuracy in defining the cardiac defect; in interventional catheterization as a palliative or curative measure; and in surgical techniques, which have led to an estimated million adults living today with complex CHD that required surgery in the neonatal period.

Despite the improvements seen in surgical correction and management of congenital heart lesions, the neurodevelopmental disabilities common in children who have cardiac defects have not decreased. As technology and surgical procedures improve and more pediatric heart surgeons use minimally invasive techniques or perform surgery on "beating" hearts, one hopes that a decrease in neurodevelopmental disabilities will be realized. Time will tell if circumventing the need for circulatory arrest during neonatal cardiac surgery leads to improved long-term outcomes. Long-term follow-up and funding for research are needed to provide the basis for evidence-based care for neonates born with congenital cardiac defects.

REFERENCES

1. Menacker F, Martin JA. Expanded health data from the new birth certificate, 2005. Natl Vital Stat Rep 2008;56(13):1–9.
2. Glickstein JS. Cardiology. In: Polin RA, Spitzer AR, editors. Fetal and neonatal secrets. Philadelphia: Elsevier Saunders; 2007. p. 80–114.
3. Knowles R, Griebsch I, Dezateux C, et al. Newborn screening for congenital heart defects: a systematic review and cost-effectiveness analysis. Health Technol Assess 2005;9(44):iii–xi.
4. Dorfman AT, Marino BS, Wernovsky G. Critical heart disease in the neonate: presentation and outcome at a tertiary center. Pediatr Crit Care Med 2008;9(3):1–10.
5. Kaplan JH, Ades AM, Rychik J. Effect of prenatal diagnosis on outcome in patient with congenital heart disease. NeoReviews 2005;6(7):e326–31.
6. Jacobs JP, Maruszewski B, European Association for Cardio-thoracic Surgery—Society of Thoracic Surgeons Joint Congenital Heart Surgery Nomenclature and Database Committee. Computerized outcomes analysis for congenital heart disease. Curr Opin Pediatr 2005;17:586–91.
7. Zannini L, Borini I. State of the art cardiac surgery in patients with congenital heart disease. J Cardiovasc Med 2007;8:3–6.
8. Onuzo OC. How effectively can clinical examination pick up congenital heart disease at birth? Arch Dis Child Fetal Neonatal Ed 2006;91:F236–7.
9. Wernovsky G, Shillingford AJ, Gaynor JW. Central nervous system outcomes in children with complex congenital heart disease. Curr Opin Cardiol 2005;20:94–9.
10. Gaynor JW, Wernovsky G. Long-term neurologic outcomes in children with congenital heart disease. In: Taeusch HW, Ballard RA, Gleason CA, editors. Avery's diseases of the newborn. Philadelphia: Elsevier Saunders; 2005. p. 896–901.
11. Kotani Y, Honjo O, Nakakura M, et al. Impact of miniaturization of cardiopulmonary bypass circuit on blood transfusion requirement in neonatal open-heart surgery. ASAIO J 2007;10:662–5.
12. Miller SP, McQuillen PS, Hamrick S, et al. Abnormal brain development in newborns with congenital heart disease. N Engl J Med 2007;357:1928–38.
13. Collins-Nakai R, McLaughlin P. How congenital heart disease originates in life. Cardiol Clin 2002;20(3):367–83.
14. Theorell C. Cardiovascular assessment of the newborn. Newborn Infant Nurs Rev 2002;2(2):111–27.
15. Park MK. Pediatric cardiology for practitioners. St. Louis (MO): Mosby; 2002.
16. Witt C. Cardiac embryology. Neonatal Netw 1997;16(1):43–9.
17. Cooper WO, Hernandez-Diaz S, Arbogast PG, et al. Major congenital malformations after first-trimester exposure to ACE inhibitors. N Engl J Med 2006;23(354):2443–51.
18. Bishara N, Clericuzio CL. Common dysmorphic syndromes in the NICU. NeoReviews 2008;3(1):e29–38.
19. Seri I, Evans J. Controversies in the diagnosis and management of hypotension in the newborn infant. Curr Opin Pediatr 2001;13(2):116–23.
20. Sansoucie DA, Cavaliere TA. Newborn and infant assessment. In: Kenner C, Lott JW, editors. Comprehensive neonatal nursing: a physiologic perspective. 3rd edition. St. Louis (MO): Saunders; 2003. p. 316–22.
21. Fleiner S. Recognition and stabilization of neonates with congenital heart disease. Newborn Infant Nurs Rev 2006;6(3):137–50.
22. Wyszynski ME. Overview of PDA pathophysiology and diagnosis. Presented at the Programs of the National Association of Neonatal Nurses Conference. San Diego (CA), September 28, 2007.
23. Killian K. Left sided obstructive congenital heart defects. Newborn Infant Nurs Rev 2006;6(3):128–36.
24. Turck CJ, Marsh W, Stevenson JG, et al. Pharmacoeconomics of surgical interventions vs. cyclooxygenase inhibitors for the treatment of patent ductus arteriosus. Journal of Pediatric Pharmacology Therapeutics 2007;12(3):183–93.
25. The Heart Institute for Children. Available at: www.thic.com. Accessed March 27, 2008.
26. American Heart Association (AHA). Surgical management of atrial septal defect. AHA News; 2008. Internet document. Available at: www.americanheart.org. Accessed January 26, 2008.
27. Lim DS, Matherne GP. Percutaneous device closure of atrial septal defect in a premature infant with rapid improvement in pulmonary status. Pediatrics 2007;119:398–400.

28. Moake L, Ramaciotti. Atrial septal defect treatment options. AACN Clin Issues 2005;16(2):252–66.
29. Jones KJ, Willis M, Uzark K. The blues of congenital heart disease. Newborn Infant Nurs Rev 2006;6(3):117–27.
30. Wernovsky G, Gruber PJ. Common congenital heart disease: presentation, management, and outcomes. In: Taeusch HW, Ballard RA, Gleason CA, editors. Avery's diseases of the newborn. 8th edition. Philadelphia: Elsevier Saunders; 2005. p. 827–71.
31. Wechsler SB, Wernovsky G. Cardiac disorders. In: Cloherty JP, Eichenwald EC, Stark AR, editors. Manual of neonatal care. 5th edition. Philadelphia: Lippincott Williams & Wilkins; 2004. p. 407–60.
32. Stein P. Total anomalous pulmonary venous connection. AORN J 2007;85(3):509–20.
33. Head CEG, Jowett VC, Sharland GK, et al. Timing of presentation and postnatal outcome of infants suspected of having coarctation of the aorta during fetal life. Heart 2005;91:1070–4.
34. Lu C, Wang J, Chang C, et al. Noninvasive diagnosis of coarctation of the aorta in neonates with patent ductus arteriosus. Pediatrics 2006;148:217–21.
35. Mayo Clinic Staff. Coarctation of the aorta. 2006. Internet document. Available at: www.mayoclinica.com. Accessed February 8, 2008.
36. Rosenthal E. Coarctation of the aorta from fetus to adult: curable condition or life long disease process? Heart 2005;91:1495–502.
37. McElhinney DB, Lock JE, Keane JF, et al. Left heart growth, function, and reintervention after balloon aortic valvuloplasty for neonatal aortic stenosis. Circulation 2005;111:451–8.
38. Weber HS, Seib PM. Aortic stenosis, valvar. eMedicine 2006. Internet document. Available at: eMedicine www.emedicine.com/PED/topic2491.htm. Accessed February 8, 2008.
39. Karamlou T, Jang K, Williams WG, et al. Outcomes and associated risk factors for aortic valve replacement in 160 children: a competing-risks analysis. Circulation 2005;112:3462–9.
40. Ahmad UA, Fatimi SH, Naqvi I, et al. Modified Blalock-Taussig shunt: immediate and short-term follow-up results. Heart Lung Circ 2007;10:10–6.
41. Chen JM, Glickstein JS, Margossian R, et al. Superior outcomes for repair in infants and neonates with tetralogy of Fallot with absent pulmonary valve syndrome. J Thorac Cardiovasc Surg 2006;132:1099–104.
42. Miatton M, De Wolf D, Francois K, et al. Intellectual, neurospsychological, and behavioral functioning in children with tetralogy of Fallot. J Thorac Cardiovasc Surg 2007;133:449–55.
43. Chamberlin M, Lozynski J. To go against nature: manipulating the neonatal ductus arteriosus with prostaglandin. Newborn Infant Nurs Rev 2006;6(3):158–64.
44. Freed DH, Robertson CM, Suave RS. Intermediate-term outcomes of the arterial switch operation for transposition of the great arteries in neonates: alive but well? J Thorac Cardiovasc Surg 2006;132(4):845–52.
45. Rasiah SV, Ewer AK, Miller P, et al. Antenatal perspectives of hypoplastic left heart syndrome: 5 years on. Arch Dis Child Fetal Neonatal Ed 2008;93:F192–7.
46. Makikallio K, McElhinney DB, Levine JC, et al. Fetal aortic valve stenosis and the evolution of hypoplastic left heart syndrome: patient selection for fetal intervention. Circulation 2006;113:1401–5.
47. Connor JA, Thiagarajan R. Hypoplastic left heart syndrome. Orphanet J Rare Dis 2007;2(23):1–5.
48. Connor JA, Thiagarajan R. Hypoplastic left heart syndrome. Neonatal Intensive Care 2008;21(1):40–3.
49. Khairy P, Poirier N, Mercier L. Univentricular heart. Circulation 2007;115:800–12.
50. Green A, Pye S, Yetman A. The physiologic basis for and nursing considerations in the use of subatmospheric concentrations of oxygen in HLHS. Adv Neonatal Care 2002;2(4):177–86.
51. Theilen U, Shekerdemian L. The intensive care of infants with hypoplastic left heart syndrome. Arch Dis Child Fetal Neonatal Ed 2005;90:F97–102.
52. Reemsten BL, Pike NA, Starnes VA. Stage I palliation for hypoplastic left heart syndrome: Norwood versus Sano modification. Curr Opin Cardiol 2007;22:60–5.
53. Li JS, Yow E, Berezny KY, et al. Clinical outcomes of palliative surgery including a systemic-to-pulmonary artery shunt in infants with cyanotic congenital heart disease: does aspirin make a difference? Circulation 2007;116:293–7.
54. Alsoufi B, Bennetts SV, Caldarone CA. New developments in the treatment of hypoplastic left heart syndrome. Pediatrics 2007;119:109–17.
55. West LJ. B-cell tolerance following ABO-incompatible infant heart transplantation. Transplantation 2006;81(3):301–7.
56. Wernovsky G, Ghanayem N, Ohye RG, et al. Hypoplastic left heart syndrome: consensus and controversies in 2007. Cardiol Young 2007;17(Suppl 2):75–86.
57. Wernovsky G, Ades AM, Spray TL. Management of congenital heart disease in the low-birth-weight infant. In: Taeusch HW, Ballard RA, Gleason CA, editors. Avery's diseases of the newborn. 8th edition. Philadelphia: Elsevier Saunders; 2005. p. 888–95.
58. Dittrich H, Buhrer C, Grimmer I. Neurodevelopment at 1 year of age in infants with congenital heart disease. Heart 2003;89:436–41.
59. Mahle WT, Visconti KJ, Freier MC, et al. Relationship of surgical approach to neurodevelopmental outcomes in hypoplastic left heart syndrome. Pediatrics 2006;117:e90–7.

60. McQuillen PS, Barkovich AJ, Hamrick SEG, et al. Temporal and anatomic risk profile of brain injury with neonatal repair of congenital heart defects. Stroke 2007;38:736–41.

61. Silva VM, Araujo TL, Lopes MVO. Evolution of nursing diagnoses for children with congenital heart disease. Rev Lat Am Enfermagem 2006;14(4):561–8.

62. Carmo KAB, Barr P, West M, et al. Transporting newborn infants with suspected duct dependent congenital heart disease on low-dose prostaglandin E1 without routine mechanical ventilation. Arch Dis Child Fetal Neonatal Ed 2007;92:F117–9.

63. Cuadrado AR. Management of postoperative low cardiac output syndrome. Crit Care Nurs Q 2002; 25(3):63–71.

64. Young TE, Mangum B. Neofax. 19th edition. Raleigh (NC): Acorn Publishing; 2006.

65. Noori S, Friedlich P, Wong P, et al. Hemodynamic changes after low-dosage hydrocortisone administration in vasopressor-treated preterm and term neonates. Pediatrics 2006;118:1456–66.

66. Piper HG, Alexander JL, Shukla A, et al. Real-time continuous glucose monitoring in pediatric patients during and after cardiac surgery. Pediatrics 2006; 118:1176–84.

67. Ward RM, Lugo RA. Pharmacologic principles and practices. In: Taeusch HW, Ballard RA, Gleason CA, editors. Avery's diseases of the newborn. 8th edition. Philadelphia: Elsevier Saunders; 2005. p. 427–37.

68. Brosig CL, Whitstone BN, Frommelt MA, et al. Psychological distress in parents of children with severe congenital heart disease: the impact of prenatal versus postnatal diagnosis. J Perinatol 2007;27(11): 687–92.

69. Upham M, Medoff-Cooper B. What are the responses & needs of mothers of infants diagnosed with congenital heart disease? MCN Am J Matern Child Nurs 2005;30(1):25–9.

70. McGrath JM, Kolwaite A. Families and chronicity of diagnosis with congenital heart defects. Newborn Infant Nurs Rev 2006;6(3):175–8.

Grass Roots Initiation of a National Certification Initiative: Peer-to-Peer Motivation

Carie E. Linder, RNC[a,b],*

KEYWORDS

- Nursing • Certification • Education
- Professional development • Motivation • Nursing staff

Although the author's institution, a large urban hospital with Magnet status, supported career ladders and advancement, in the neonatal ICU (NICU), few nurses held national specialty certification. To rectify this situation, a peer-to-peer mentor program was started. Its express purpose was to increase the empowerment of NICU nurses and to advance the number of certified nurses. This article describes the grass roots initiation of this program and discusses the outcomes in relation to NICU certification achievements of the nursing staff.

MOTIVATION TO EXCEL

The hospital's philosophy of maintaining Magnet status and the emphasis on being the best nurse possible influenced the author's NICU to encourage nurses to obtain national certification. To begin this process, one nurse had to take the lead. The influence of change can be initiated by the act of a single individual; however, the process is entrenched in the psychology of motivation, crucial organization, and provision of ample support and recognition. This certification program was developed parallel to the author's own certification process, who assumed the roles of developer and participant at the program's start. Inspiration for this program originated from the independent success of one nurse, one mentor.

Obtaining a national certification in a clinical specialty elevates the nurse professionally and personally. Attainment of this goal engages the nurse in the profession, identifying the nurse as a leader, role model, and mentor. The process of certification is not a final goal; instead, it is the opportunity to immerse oneself in the nursing profession. Nursing is perpetually evolving, and acceptance of this professional role includes the understanding that engagement in lifelong learning is essential to maintain skills and knowledge. The certified nurse embraces this commitment of an educational continuum.

THE GRASS ROOTS PROGRAM

The process of motivating nurses to pursue this goal has remained elusive. The Grass Roots program was developed as a support network, providing nurses with the tools needed to ensure success on their certification examination. The program's focus is to motivate and cultivate an optimistic mindset by way of structure and support, establishing certification as an obtainable and desirable goal. The certification process can be confusing and overwhelming, often presenting a preliminary barrier to goal attainment.

CERTIFICATION

Numerous benefits of certification attainment—from the prospective of nurses, management, and

This work was supported in part by the nonprofit organization Neonatal Quality Initiative Network (NQIN) developed by Edward Co, MD.
[a] Neonatal Intensive Care Unit, Integris Baptist Medical Center, Oklahoma City, OK, USA
[b] University of Oklahoma Health Science Center, College of Nursing, Oklahoma City, OK, USA
* Corresponding author. University of Oklahoma Health Science Center, College of Nursing, PO Box 26901, Oklahoma City, OK 73126
E-mail address: carie.linder@integris-health.com

Crit Care Nurs Clin N Am 21 (2009) 49–55
doi:10.1016/j.ccell.2008.10.002

patients—have been explored and identified within the literature. Obtaining a national certification provides nurses with an opportunity to be recognized and valued for an advanced level of achievement. Successful examination validates the nurse's specialty knowledge, expertise, and judgment, providing a benchmark of credentialing excellence.[1] A certified nurse can quantitatively measure success and knowledge comparatively across the nation. Examinees must meet professional requirements in the area of specialty or clinical practice and meet eligibility requirements that include minimum hourly direct bedside or specialty nursing care.[1,2]

A survey by the American Board of Nursing Specialties (ABNS) identified that certified and noncertified nurses perceive the benefits of obtaining certification as including the ability to enhance professional autonomy, identify clinical competency, and enhance personal confidence in clinical abilities.[3] Certification empowers nurses to be confident in their abilities to achieve excellence, provide the highest quality nursing care, and improve medical knowledge and clinical skills. These factors influence the nurse's perception of power and autonomy, which improves nursing job satisfaction and enhances retention.[1]

Within the health care consumer culture, the public acknowledges the value of national certification and demonstrates a preference for hospitals that have a higher percentage of certified nurses.[1] One of the focuses for the award of Magnet status by the American Nurses Credentialing Center (ANCC) is expanding professional development. Within hospitals receiving this recognition, 26% of all nursing staff is nationally certified in their area of specialty.[4]

Preceding the launch of this program, a dialogue was introduced to the unit staff that identified hindering factors related to pursuing certification. A retrospective comparison found that the results were surprisingly similar to barriers to certification identified by the 2006 ABNS survey.[3] The nurses within the unit most often cited factors revolving around financial investment of examination fees and study materials, confusion over the application process, lack of identified institutional value, anxiety over examination, and lack of study time and skills. The unit staff further expressed confusion about the selection of an appropriate certification, the identification of study materials, and the burden of mandatory continuing nursing education (CNE) requirements for certification maintenance. Oklahoma does not have an annual CNE requirement for nursing license maintenance.[5]

Currently, there are over 40 professional nursing organizations that provide nationally recognized certification in specialty areas. These organizations offer approximately 135 certifications in various clinical and nonclinical specialties of nursing.[6,7] The question then moves from "Should I certify?" to "Which certification should I pursue?" Occasionally, there are overlapping certifications offered by separate organizations. When determining what certification is most appropriate, one should first look at specialized professional organizations: do they have an embedded certification or a program with which they have become aligned? Participants should assess the organization's mission statement to determine whether it is congruent with their beliefs and reflective of the highest nursing standards. Another question that should be addressed is whether the certification is recognized as the gold standard.

It is important for potential participants to examine each organization, converse with peers, and explore which certification is best for their advancement. Currently, the NICU specialty certification offered by the National Certification Corporation (NCC) is High-Risk Neonatal Nursing. The nurse who successfully passes the certification examination has the privilege of using the RNC (registered nurse, certified) credential. The American Association of Critical-Care Nurses (AACN) Certification Corporation has traditionally credentialed nurses who successfully complete the examination as a critical-care registered nurse (CCRN).

The author has maintained a professional alliance as a member of the AACN for several years; however, the nursing culture of the author's institution identifies most with the certification provided by the NCC. The historical cultural alliance is with the NCC, a not-for-profit organization that provides the credentialing programs for nurses, physicians, and other licensed health care personnel.[2] This recognition provided the final decision of which certification to pursue. Because this decision is a possible point of divergence, each candidate must weigh outcome benefits. With the benefits of certification identified and the perceived hindrances eliminated, what would prevent registered nurses from becoming nationally certified?

THE PARTICIPANTS

The program's unit is a 28-bed level III NICU within a metropolitan teaching Magnet hospital. The participants averaged 11 years of nursing practice within this specific NICU. The participants' mean age was 39 years, with multiple occurrence of a 3-decade variance. Many nurses had identified "obtaining a national certification" as a professional goal on their annual evaluations; however, this goal was perceived as unobtainable due to overwhelming hindering factors such as time, money, and lack of confidence in passing the examination.

A SUCCESSFUL PROGRAM

A peer-to-peer program was developed to personally motivate, support, and encourage participation in the process of certification. Seven phases of the program were identified: initiation, promotion, support, surprise, recognition, follow-through, and peer pressure. A vital feature of this program was the peer coordinator. The author served as the program's peer coordinator, whose role was that of a facilitator and a resource for each participant at every phase of the program.

Initiation

The program was initiated with the development of a unit-based certification committee. The members executed a detailed needs assessment that explored unit-specific issues. The committee identified issues related to perceived hindering factors, motivational rewards, and desired recognition methods. At this point, the type of certification to pursue was investigated and the selection was made. The committee was responsible for identifying financial, educational, and managerial resources available for program development, support, and implementation.

Identification of resources: educational

The first task the committee embarked on was to explore the literature currently available in the market. The Grass Roots program chose the NCC certifying body for certification examination. It is unfortunate that recommended materials are not clearly identified or provided by this organization, requiring an extensive investigation outside the scope of the certifying body. Ironically, a well-developed and organized resource for a self-directed study was developed for the AACN certification program. Accurate identification of educational resources required for success is essential for the second phase of initiation.

Identification of resources: financial

The next phase of program development was clear identification and communication of financial needs. Exploration of alternate funding methods and opportunities for cost sharing with participants should be identified before management is approached. The program received complete financial support from the institution in collaboration with a grant from the Neonatal Quality Initiative Network (NQIN).

The unit needs assessment identified the financial burden of examination fees and study resources as a primary barrier to certification. During the development of the program, the hospital offered an examination-fee reimbursement program, providing full reimbursement of examination fees on successful certification. Many nurses did not access this resource and expressed anxiety and hesitation related to the perceived gamble and potential loss of income. The program goal, however, was to eliminate all financial responsibilities for the examination candidate, eradicating barriers and diminishing anxieties.

A grant application was submitted to Edward Co, MD, president and founder of NQIN, an attending Pediatrix neonatologist within the author's institution. The Grass Roots program and the NQIN formally established a partnership with the long-term goal of developing and promoting quality initiatives in the areas of clinical improvement and nursing education that would result in improved neonatal outcomes. This focus is congruent with the vision of the NQIN, a nonprofit network that is working to achieve excellence in quality neonatal care.[8]

In an effort to eliminate the primary barrier of examination fees, the concept of an examination-fee scholarship program was initiated. The development of a culture of certification was concurrent with the hospital system's initial application for consideration for Magnet status, which was obtained during the program's inception. The hospital system simultaneously developed a National Certification Examination Fee Assistance Program that provided a full examination-fee scholarship for two specialty certifications for each employee. This incentive addressed and alleviated the primary inhibiting factors. Furthermore, the organization implemented a $1000 primary bonus and an Annual Bonus Incentive Program that provides an additional $1000 bonus each year for the maintenance of certification.

The NQIN granted permission to redirect grant funds for the establishment of a certification library. The coordinator developed a cost analysis for the certification program. The analysis identified items that would be required for 10 participants to enter to the certification program and for the establishment of the certification library. These items consisted of core curriculum text, practice examinations, practice questions, and a video certification review program. The study items would be on loan from the unit and, on completion of the program, would be returned to the coordinator for loan to the next certification group. The committee identified an opportunity for cost sharing with participants, requesting individuals to purchase the corresponding syllabus compatible with the video certification series. The syllabus would provide each participant with an additional 16 CNE credits.

A retrospective assessment of the incentives and the recognition of certification incorporated into this program showed concurrent integration of numerous incentives identified by the ABNS survey.[3] Additional direct financial incentives provided to the participants included 8 hours of paid training time for an approved preparation course and an additional 16 hours of paid training for annual continuing education.

Identification of resources: managerial

System-wide managerial buy-in is essential. More than just a financial resource, the physical presence of and acknowledgment from all levels of management validate the importance of certification and the investment in staff development. Managerial support in the certification process is meaningful to the nurse, much more than perceived by management. Managerial and physician support demonstrates a unified goal of increased nursing autonomy and education advancement.[1]

Promotion

The third phase of this program focused on generating staff interest, excitement, and enthusiasm and encouraging participation in the program. Initial promotion of the program was expressed in a full-color 4 ft × 3 ft conceptualization poster entitled "RNC in 3." The poster was hung at the employee entrance to the unit. The information conveyed included identification of rewards and incentives, clear explanation of expectations, timelines, examination topics, financial incentives, identification of support, and supplies provided by the program.

Alongside this announcement poster was a posted sign-up sheet limited to 10 participants. The method of public acknowledgment and acceptance of the challenge of obtaining RNC certification in 3 months obligated participant accountability. The process of asking each participant to openly and publicly accept this challenge generated encouragement and support from peers and team members.

After the participants were identified, a detailed process map was developed and posted (**Fig. 1**). The poster was laminated and exaggerated in size and color. A large red "you are here" arrow was used to identify the current stage of the certification process. At each point of advancement, the poster was updated to reflect goal achievement and to keep the participants on track.

Support

The program coordinator serves as the primary support and resource for participants. The coordinator must be informed, organized, and accessible. This role is not that of an educator but a facilitator. After participants were identified, NICU certification packets were developed and distributed. Each packet contained an examination processes poster, a three-page study calendar, an application for examination, a fact and information sheet, a directory for support including Web site addresses, additional study resources, step-by-step guidance for identification of testing sites with a full-color map, and documents needed for accessing the examination-fee assistance and bonus. Each participant received a copy of a course review textbook, practice questions with rationale, and a practice examination. The calendar study guide was developed to provide each participant with clearly defined week-by-week course reading selections and corresponding practice questions. The course review was organized to commence, progress, and conclude within a 12-week period. The course review was independent study. The self-directed learning format is cost-effective, consistent with information delivery, convenient, and readily available.[9]

During the last month of study, the coordinator organized a group activity using a multimedia course review purchased from AACN. Management demonstrated its support of participants and acknowledged their efforts by relieving participants of their schedule obligations. Participants received paid educational time for attendance, comfortable amenities away from the unit, and provisions during the course. Such select privileges promote the spirit of learning and elevate the value of the certification process by demonstrating managerial commitment.[9]

Surprise

The certification committee recognized and supported each participant's commitment by delivering a "care package" to his or her home. The contents included a fun note from the certification committee, encouraging the participants in their studies. The care package contained highlighters, pens, snacks, powdered drink, and fun cup. These packages were creative and unique for each participant group. The committee received an overwhelming response of surprise, gratitude, and appreciation from participants, demonstrating that just a little extra effort served to reinforce and acknowledge the participants' hard work.

Recognition

Individual, appropriate, and sincere recognition of goal attainment is essential for program success. This program celebrated with a private certification

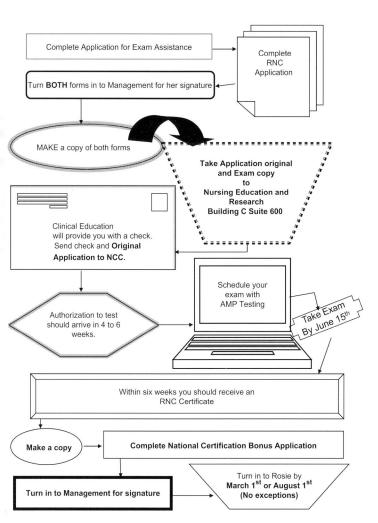

Fig. 1. An RNC examination application process map identifying stages and timelines for the certification process.

luncheon for participants, clinical managers, unit directors, unit physicians, and members of upper management. The celebration provided an opportunity for a public acknowledgement of the participants' goal attainment. Each participant was independently recognized and presented with an institution-developed certificate of achievement. The participant's name was added to the NICU's certification plaque displaying the unit's certified nurses. The luncheon was another opportunity to identify certification as a goal that is valued system wide and to demonstrate managerial support. A color photo of the participant recognition ceremony appeared in the institution's quarterly newsletter. An annual recognition luncheon exclusive to certified nurses is in development.

Follow-Through

The goal in the development of Grass Roots was to eliminate all barriers to certification. The final barriers identified by the staff were the certification

maintenance requirements and the lack of post-certification CNE opportunities. For this type of program to be successful, follow-through must be as important as initiation. The hospital system provides an annual bonus of $1000 for certification maintenance, which demonstrates a long-term commitment from management to assist with continuing education and renewal fees. To demonstrate that certification is not just the final goal but the first step in the nurses' reinvestment in knowledge acquisition and increased autonomy, increased on-campus CNE opportunities need to be investigated and initiated, with a communication board used to share resources for free CNEs offered online or in print.

Peer Pressure

Singling out and promoting the unit's certified nurses provided an unintended level of peer pressure—a paradigm shift in the unit's expectations. A cohesive group has developed that supports each member throughout the process of certification. Nurses who have earned their certification become mentors, empathizing with the next round of participants and recognizing their successes. Certification becomes a team building process, instigated and supported by peers.

A change in expectations has been established with the new nursing graduates. They are introduced to the units' culture of certification with the expectation of initiating the certification process at the point of qualification. This is the essence of a culture of certification—the process is supported and valued by all members. The development of this program and its success has been promoted within the hospital facility, setting new expectations for other units.

DISCUSSION

There were many areas during the development and implementation of the program that required modification or abandonment. The development of an extended certification committee did not become a reality, primarily due to scheduling conflicts and limited initial interest. Responsibility of the program and implementation resided with the coordinator and with Edward Co, MD.

Originally, consideration of weekly or biweekly study groups was considered. Due to scheduling conflicts, this concept was abandoned but was replaced with the self-directed learning modules purchased from the professional organization. The self-directed learning style proved to be most successful because of convenience and the fact that learning occurs at an individual pace.

Other issues arose from learning modules used for the certification. The AACN materials were chosen because of their encompassing information and organization; however, the video review program, which combined pediatric and neonatal material, proved to be very distracting and overwhelming to the first participant group. The experience and examination of the first participant group (including that of the coordinator) allowed for a more tailored and focused review in future sessions.

Ideally, this unit strives for 100% certification; however, certification presented as a mandatory process nullifies the concept of independent knowledge acquisition and empowerment. The process of certification must be independently initiated and not imposed by management. The process embodies the participants' commitment and dedication to the profession of nursing. Participants must be self-motivated and goal oriented. When certification is imposed as a requirement, it manifests resentment and resistance and becomes a burden.

As the coordinator, it is important to identify nurses who have learning differences, difficulties, and excessive anxieties related to testing. These participants require special consideration and modifications to the program. Exploring alternate texts, multimedia enhancements, or secondary sources of information may be required. The coordinator must openly and compassionately address participants' fears and frustrations.

Public acknowledgement and acceptance of challenge thrived in this unit, but considerations should be made for those individuals uncomfortable with the examination process. The goal is to minimize anxieties, not induce them.

Initially, the program was criticized for "spoon feeding" the staff with all of the required information, forms, and texts at no cost. There were concerns that the participants would take advantage of the program and not reciprocate with the investment of study required for success. Additional apprehension related to individuals accepting financial assistance and depleting finds without benefit or replenishment was discussed. The use of public acknowledgment of acceptance into the program provided adequate accountability.

Review of the original needs assessment identified many barriers to obtaining certification. This program eliminated all barriers identified except study time and anxiety. The role of the coordinator is to minimize anxiety with organization, insight, study tools, and information.

RESULTS

At completion of this first year, the goal of increasing the percentage of nationally certified nurses was achieved. The first year of the certification program yielded a 38% unit increase in certified nurses. The institution's unit total of eligible certified neonatal nurses is now calculated at 59%, well above the national average. The program has established a 100% participant success rate on the certification examination.

Unintended Consequences

The program was embraced by the staff, management, and physicians and facilitated a realignment of unit expectations. New graduates are encouraged to begin study and to use the core curriculum from onset of orientation to familiarize themselves with the material and concepts. Examination at point of qualification is the unit expectation. Evidence of nursing empowerment has been demonstrated by the commencement of the first nurse-initiated research study within the unit. The certification process has been integrated into career advancement by becoming a prerequisite for participation in the transport team.

The unit experienced a decline, more appropriately described as an abruption in turnover: not a single full-time nurse has resigned from the NICU since the initiation of the RNC program. Research has shown that certified nurses perceive a deeper level of empowerment in their profession and experience a new level of respect from management and peers.[5] The establishment of this program and its success has enhanced recruitment for an expanding unit and has become a promotional tool. The hospital management and NQIN invested in the staff by offering financial incentives and grants to stimulate and promote higher education and by providing emotional support to demonstrate appreciation and improve morale. Observed benefits of this certification process are the increased knowledge and clinical skills demonstrated by the certified nurses and their increased participation in clinical improvement programs. Through the CNE requirements, the staff is up-to-date on current research and evidence-based medicine.

The program success has not been confined to the NICU—the process has expanded to the newborn nursery and outlying facilities. Currently, satellite programs are being established in other hospitals. The unique opportunity for expansion of this program to other units outside the author's institution further augments the program's goal. Sharing this program's concepts and success can only benefit the true stakeholders: our patients.

SUMMARY

Even though the benefits to certification have been identified and validated; inhibiting factors and motivational tools from the nursing perspective have been explored and acknowledged; and the body of literature, resources, and professional organizations supporting the process of certification is abundant, the process of developing a culture of certification has remained elusive for many medical centers.

The parallel roles of program developer, peer coordinator, and participant provided the author with unique perspectives that provided insight into participant fears, concerns, motivation, and reward. The peer-to-peer relationship facilitated partnership and camaraderie throughout the certification process. The Grass Roots program incorporated multiple perspectives, integrated information, and developed a successful program process of promotion, facilitation, and recognition.

This program demonstrates how the influence of change can be initiated by the act of a single individual.

ACKNOWLEDGMENTS

The author would like to thank Edward Co, MD, for his unwavering support and motivation with this project and his commitment to nursing education and advancement; Carole Kenner, DNS, RNC-NIC, FAAN, Dean of the College of Nursing, University of Oklahoma Health Science Center, for her guidance, editing, and support; M.J. Linder for her editorial assistance throughout the program; and LaTonya Sango RNC, mentor and unintentional initiator of change.

Perpetual gratitude goes to the nursing staff of Integris Baptist Medical Center Neonatal Intensive Care Unit, Oklahoma City, Oklahoma, for their encouragement, dedication, and many accomplishments. They are integral to the tremendous success of this program.

REFERENCES

1. American Association of Critical-Care Nurses. Certification. Available at: http://www.aacn.org. 2008; Accessed on June 15, 2008.
2. American Nurses Credentialing Center. Why AACN certification? Available at: http://www.nursecredentialing.org. 2008; Accessed on June 15, 2008.
3. American Board of Nursing Specialties. Specialty nursing certification: nurses' perceptions, values and behaviors. Available at: http://www.nursingcertification.org/pdf/white_paper_final_12_12_06_pdf. 2006; Accessed on June 7, 2008.
4. American Nurses Credentialing Center. Magnet Recognition Program. Available at: http://ancc.com. 2008; Accessed on June 12, 2008.
5. Oklahoma State Board of Nursing. Requirements for registration and renewal as a registered nurse. Available at: http://www.state.ok.us/nursing/rules07.pdf. 2008; Accessed on June 22, 2008.
6. Your Guide to Certification. AJN Career Guide 2008. Am J Nurs 2008;108:69–70.
7. Wolf P. Career directory. Specialty certification organizations. Nursing 2008;33:20–1.
8. Neonatal Quality Initiative Network. NQIN: working together to achieve excellence in quality neonatal care [brochure]. Available at: http://www.neonatalquality.org. 2008; Accessed January 2008.
9. Trapp P. Engaging the body and mind with the spirit of learning to promote critical thinking. J Contin Educ Nurs 2005;36(2):73–6.

Gently Caring: Supporting the First Few Critical Hours of Life for the Extremely Low Birth Weight Infant

Dianne S. Charsha, RN, MSN, NNP-BC

KEYWORDS

- Extremely low birth weight infant (ELBW)
- ELBW stabilization • ELBW resuscitationm
- ELBW parent support

Infants who are born weighing less than 2500 g are classified as low birth weight (LBW) infants; very low birth weight (VLBW) infants weigh less than 1500 g, but extremely low birth weight (ELBW) infants weigh less than 1000 g and are usually born at less than 28 weeks' gestation. Unfortunately, 1 in 10 infants born with low birth weight are in the ELBW category. ELBW survival has improved over the past 20 years with the use of maternal steroids and surfactant administration. The minimum age of viability is now 23 weeks' gestation with a few surviving at 21 and 22 weeks' gestation. Mortality and morbidity rises as gestational age decreases.[1]

CAUSE

Infants are born prematurely for many reasons. Prenatal risk factors leading to premature birth are many and are listed under the following categories:

- Predisposing maternal factors: socioeconomic status, nutritional state, age, and drug use, stress, and so forth
- Pre-existing medical conditions: diabetes, hypertension, thyroid disorders, anemia, cardiac compromise, systemic lupus erythematosis, and so forth
- Obstetric issues: habitual aborter, blood group sensitization, history of stillborn,

infection, placental or cord issues, multiple gestations, pre-eclampsia/eclampsia
- Fetal complications: chromosomal, anatomic abnormality, position

MINIMIZING PREMATURE BIRTH

Unfortunately, the leading cause of prematurity is still a mystery. Therefore, a tremendous effort is being made to provide and encourage prenatal care for all pregnant women. The earlier prenatal care is initiated, the earlier testing can be performed and interventions started to improve outcome. Lifestyle issues are repeatedly addressed during these visits and advice for improving health is reinforced. During prenatal care, the woman is educated about the signs and symptoms of preterm labor, other complications, and when to seek medical attention. Signs of preterm labor include

Abdominal cramping
Increase in vaginal discharge
Low intermittent or continuous backache
Pelvic pressure[2]

In many cases, premature labor identified early can be stopped with hydration, rest, treating an underlying infection, or administration of a tocolytic. Tocolytics may be selected to stop preterm labor if

Uterine contractions are causing cervical dilatation or effacement

Cooper University Hospital, Nursing Administration #213, One Cooper Plaza, Camden, NJ 08103, USA
E-mail address: charsha-dianne@cooperhealth.edu

Crit Care Nurs Clin N Am 21 (2009) 57–65
doi:10.1016/j.ccell.2008.09.003
0899-5885/08/$ – see front matter © 2009 Elsevier Inc. All rights reserved.

Fetus is premature and lungs are immature (amniotic fluid analyses: lecithin/sphingo-myelin ratio, phosphatidyl glycerol, and optical density 650)[3]

Maternal status is healthy

If premature birth is unavoidable or anticipated before 34 weeks' gestation, maternal steroids should be considered to optimize fetal lung maturity. The following indications may necessitate an extremely premature delivery:

Acute fetal distress
Chorioamnionitis
Severe pre-eclampsia or eclampsia
Severe fetal growth restriction
Maternal physiologic instability[4]

Depending on the institution's maternal or neonatal capability, the mother or neonate may need to be transported to a higher level of care.

COMPLICATIONS OF PREMATURITY

The complications of prematurity are many, especially with decreasing gestational age. The following disorders are of significant importance to the overall outcome of the smallest infants.

Intraventricular Hemorrhage

Intraventricular hemorrhage (IVH) is an intracranial hemorrhage that occurs in the highly vascular periventricular germinal matrix area and can extend into the ventricular system and out into the parenchyma. The incidence of IVH has fallen to below 20% but 90% of the bleeds occur during the first 3 days of life and ELBW infants are at greatest risk.[5] Other risk factors for IVH include asphyxia, resuscitation, ventilation, pneumothorax, rapid administration of hypertonic drugs, or sudden change in blood pressure. The Papile IVH classification system is shown in **Box 1**.

Signs and symptoms of IVH include apnea, bradycardia, anemia, acidosis, seizures, bulging fontanel, shock, change in level of consciousness, or they can be completely asymptomatic.

Diagnosis is usually made by a neural ultrasound and is usually acquired by a week to 10 days of life for infants at risk for IVH. The greater the stage of the bleed, the more likely that neurologic sequelae will occur.

Periventricular Leukomalacia

Periventricular leukomalacia (PVL) is hypoxic-ischemic necrosis of the periventricular white matter. It can occur with or without IVH. The incidence of PVL increases with decreasing gestational age. Asphyxia or a decrease in cerebral blood flow are the primary causes of PVL and these events can occur around the time of birth. Because PVL results in a loss of brain tissue, it is usually diagnosed by a neural ultrasound or MRI performed at least 30 days following a birth. PVL seen on neural ultrasound at 1 week of life usually indicates an old event in utero. PVL can result in cerebral palsy.

Retinopathy of Prematurity

Retinopathy of prematurity (ROP) is a disruption in the vascularization of the developing retina. ROP is most commonly noted with decreasing gestational age. ROP represents 20% of blindness in preschool children.[7] Vessels on the retina start to develop at about 16 weeks' gestation on the nasal side of the retina and progress across the surface to the temporal side around term. Elevated oxygen levels and a complex neonatal course can lead to ROP. ROP is evaluated by stages, as shown in **Box 2**.

Plus disease may occur during stages 2 to 4 when vessels posterior to the ridge become dilated and tortuous.[8]

The more advanced the ROP stage, the worse the prognosis, and plus disease is never a good

---

Box 1
Papile intraventricular hemorrhage classification system

Grade 1: Germinal matrix hemorrhage

Grade 2: IVH without ventricular dilatation

Grade 3: IVH with ventricular dilatation

Grade 4: Germinal matrix or IVH hemorrhage with parenchymal involvement[6]

Box 2
International classification of retinopathy of prematurity

Stage 1: Thin demarcation line between the vascularized region of the retina and the avascular zone

Stage 2: The demarcation line develops into a ridge protruding into the vitreous

Stage 3: Extraretinal fibrovascular proliferation occurs on the ridge

Stage 4: Neovascularization extends into the vitreous, causing traction on the retina, resulting in subtotal retinal detachment

Stage 5: Total retinal detachment

diagnosis. Eye examinations are usually performed at 4 to 6 weeks of age or around 32 weeks postconceptual age. These examinations are periodically continued until intervention is indicated or a mature retina is assessed. Cryoplexy or laser surgery can be performed to try to stop the progression of the disease.

Hearing Deficit

Hearing deficit may be caused by medical administration of ototoxic drugs required during the neonatal course (ie, furosemide, aminoglycosides) or by a central neurologic deficit like an IVH or PVL. Therefore, all infants being discharged from the newborn intensive care unit (NICU) should have a baseline hearing screen assessment. Early detection of hearing loss enables intervention, which may enhance the infant's ability to meet language developmental milestones.

Bronchopulmonary Dysplasia

Bronchopulmonary dysplasia (BPD) is the neonatal form of chronic lung disease and usually results from an extended period of ventilation or prolonged oxygen requirement. BPD is defined by an oxygen need that persists beyond 36 weeks postconceptual age. Infants born prematurely have immature lungs. Maternal steroid administration helps enhance lung maturity and surfactant production. The incidence of BPD increases with decreasing gestational age. The major contributing factors leading to BPD are oxygen exposure, mechanical ventilation, and inflammation, which usually start in the first few days of life. BPD is best prevented by preventing premature birth or treating respiratory distress syndrome with surfactant as indicated. It is a priority to administer only the ventilatory assistance required to support adequate oxygenation and ventilation. Care of the infant who has BPD is supportive.

Necrotizing Enterocolitis

Necrotizing enterocolitis (NEC) results from an injured immature gastrointestinal system so it is predominately a disorder of premature infants. Asphyxia, inadequate perfusion, and enteral feedings are commonly identified in the history of neonates who have NEC. Like all the other complications of prematurity, the incidence of NEC increases with decreasing gestational age. NEC is also staged like many of the neonatal complications. See **Box 3**.

Diagnosis is usually made by identifying pneumatosis, intrahepatic portal venous gas, or free air by radiograph. Treatment of NEC usually includes supportive management: nothing by mouth

---

Box 3
Stages of necrotizing enterocolitis
Stage 1: Suspected NEC (feeding intolerance, guaiac-positive stools)
Stage 2a: Ileus, dilated loops, some pneumatosis intestinalis on radiograph (H+ gas in bowel lining outlines the bowel on radiograph)
Stage 2b: Extensive pneumatosis intestinalis, intrahepatic portal venous gas
Stage 3a: Prominent ascites, paucity of bowel gas
Stage 3b: Absent bowel gas, evidence of intraperitoneal free air[9]

(NPO), nasogastric tube to suction, support and monitoring of total body functions, antibiotics, and frequent laboratory and radiograph monitoring. Surgical intervention is indicated when free air is noted or when the child is not improving with supportive medical management. Necrotic bowel can make the child present with acidosis, shock, or progressive leukopenia, granulocytopenia, and thrombocytopenia.

So, being born at less than 1000 g and before 28 weeks' gestation has significant risks for mortality and morbidity. These children should be born, when possible, in a center that is extremely experienced in the care of these neonates.

EXTREMELY LOW BIRTH WEIGHT OVERVIEW

As we test the limits of viability, it is critical that we integrate a protective and developmentally supportive approach to the actual resuscitation and stabilization aspects of care to provide maximal protection to the brain and central nervous system. To achieve this goal, we must provide coordinated, comprehensive, experienced, and supportive care to the ELBW infant.

At every step during resuscitation and stabilization, we should communicate and partner with the parents, involving them in the decision making and offering choices when possible. The health care team should review common complications of the ELBW infant, along with treatment options. Full disclosure is vital to ensure that the parents fully understand the condition and potential prognosis of their infant. To help parents make the best decisions for their family, each facility should consider sharing its center's experience with the various birth weights and gestational age groups. Information that might be helpful would include mortality rates, along with critical morbidity statistics such as IVH, PVL, surgical NEC, and surgical ROP.

It is always preferable to deliver the ELBW infant in a tertiary care center where perinatal and neonatal services are readily available.[10] An ELBW infant requiring transport in the first few days of life is at increased risk for complications.[11]

PREPARATION

If time permits, the parents or family should be told what to expect in the infant's first few hours after birth. When viability is in question, the decision points or questions that they might be asked soon after delivery should be explained. If the birth precedes parent preparation (timing, illness, and so forth), decisions can always be made at a later point when the infant is in the NICU.

The importance of preparing the delivery room and the neonatal team for the birth of an ELBW infant cannot be overemphasized. Having an ELBW delivery room protocol can help facilitate preparation efforts. It is important for every person in the delivery room to have an identified role during the resuscitation (airway/direction, vital signs/chest compressions, respiratory and monitoring equipment, and medication/documentation). Having too many care providers in the delivery room can cause crowding and potential confusion.

The delivery room should be prewarmed when possible, along with the stabilization area if separate, to 25° to 28°C or 77° to 82.4°F.[12] Rooms used to deliver/stabilize ELBW infants should be free from drafts around the neonatal bed area. Air deflectors can be helpful when drafts are noted. A neonatal delivery warmer and NICU admission bed should always be warm for the next delivery/admission,[13] with warmed blankets readily available. Beds are on the market that can serve as warmers/incubators and transport vehicles. Each center needs to evaluate its selection of bed devices to determine which equipment choice will optimize thermal support for the ELBW infant in its institution's setting. It is optimal to have a bed scale on the stabilization warmer to avoid additional cold stress. A chemical mattress can be used to aid in maintaining the infant's temperature but must be activated just before the birth.[14] If using a chemical mattress, one should check the manufacturer's recommendations about placing a light sheet over the mattress before use and its maximum duration of thermal support. Some mattresses become cool past their useful life and can actually remove heat from the infant. A warmed, U-shaped towel roll can be placed on a warmed blanket over the chemical mattress to aid extremity flexion and thermal support. If a transporter is

going to be used to transport the infant to the NICU, it must also be prepared and warmed.[15]

Blended oxygen should be available to the ELBW infant in the delivery room,[13] along with a device to provide positive pressure ventilation. Many centers are placing ELBW infants directly on a continuous positive airway pressure (CPAP) device or ventilator to avoid variable pressures administered by hand-held bag devices. This equipment needs to be set up and functional at the time of delivery.

RESUSCITATION

On delivery of the ELBW infant, the physician should clamp and cut the cord while the other physician or first assistant blots the infant's skin of amniotic fluid and places him/her feet first into a sterile plastic bag up to his/her neck. This bag helps reduce convective and evaporative heat loss during the transfer to the warmer and during the resuscitation, because vigorous drying of the infant to prevent hypothermia is not possible with the ELBW infant's fragile skin.[15] It is optimal for the individual receiving the infant from the delivery table to have a preheated sterile towel in hand to receive the infant. The bed scale can be zeroed before placing the infant down on the bed so that a quick weight can be obtained at the time the infant is placed on the mattress, which will avoid further movement, handling, and potential cold stress. At this point, a loose-fitting hat, which can be the traditional term delivery room cap, should be placed on the head to avoid further heat loss. An alternative hat used to secure a CPAP apparatus or to keep a bilirubin mask in place can also be chosen.

Whenever possible, the infant's head should be maintained in a midline and slightly elevated position. The elevated position can be maintained by tipping up the foot of the bed and placing the infant's head at the foot for easy airway access for the resuscitation team. Midline head position can be maintained in a supine, right-, or left-sided position, depending on the alignment of the body. Research has shown that cerebral blood flow is altered when the newborn head is not kept midline and elevated.[16] This position is usually maintained during the most at-risk period for IVH (before 96 hours of age).[17]

Oxygen can be started around 30% to 40% fraction of inspired oxygen (FIO_2) and titrated to acquire a centrally pink color or until the pulse oximeter indicates an 85% to 95% saturation.[18] Ventilation and oxygenation can be supported with CPAP or mechanical ventilation, as required. It is always preferable to offer only the level of support required by the infant. If mechanical ventilation is indicated, then intubation should be performed by the most experienced individual present and surfactant administered when the infant has a stable heart rate and is centrally pink, with a pulse oximeter applied.[19] Prewarming the surfactant to room or body temperature or per the manufacturer's recommendations can aid in its spread and avoid further cooling of the infant. Whenever possible, a pulse oximeter should be used to monitor oxygenation during surfactant administration.[20] This oximeter will also help monitor heart rate and oxygenation during the infant's transfer from bed to transporter or from delivery room to NICU.

STABILIZATION

Once admitted to the NICU, the ELBW infant should be assigned to an experienced nurse and respiratory therapist who are familiar with the stabilization and needs of this fragile population. The infant can be supported with his/her head on a flat gel pillow to dissipate pressure across the scalp surface and support the relatively large head. These pillows also help minimize head molding and facilitate a more rounded head shape.[21] Because the infant has a large occiput, a small roll placed under his/her shoulders can help maintain his/her airway in an optimal sniffing position. U-shaped boundaries should be maintained around the infant to maintain his/her extremities in a flexed position, with knees and hands supported toward midline.

It is to be hoped that the supportive thermal measures taken in the delivery room have maintained the infant's temperature above 36°C[22] when the infant is admitted to the NICU and removed from the plastic bag covering his/her trunk and extremities. Tracking the NICU admission temperatures of the ELBW infant, striving to keep the temperature between 36°C and 37°C, is an excellent performance improvement project for the neonatal tertiary care setting. The warmer/incubator temperature probe should be placed on the infant's abdomen, away from the umbilicus and any bony prominence, with a hydrogel-backed reflective shield to protect the skin from epidermal stripping.[23] Pectin or hydrocolloid barriers, such as extrathin duoderm, can be used on either side of the probe as a supportive base to secure the reflective shield on extremely premature thin skin.[24] A heating mattress can be used to maintain or enhance thermal support when a warmer or incubator is inadequate to meet the needs of a specific infant. Shields or saran can be used to minimize evaporative or convective thermal losses.[25] It is optimal to keep this device or material away from the infant's skin to avoid friction injury.

The infant's vital functions should be reassessed on admission. To aid the skin integrity of the extremely premature infant, heart rate can be monitored continuously by way of an arterial line or from the pulse oximeter. When used, monitor leads should be backed with hydrogel and sized for the ELBW infant. Limb leads may be chosen to avoid artifact on chest and abdominal radiographs or when an inadequate surface area or intact skin is not available for traditional chest and abdominal lead placement. Sponge wraps can secure pulse oximeter probes without the use of adhesive.

Oxygen administration should be adjusted to maintain saturation levels at between 85% and 95%. Breath sounds should be bilaterally equal, with a slight chest rise/expansion noted. If the infant is on a ventilator and has received surfactant, tidal volumes should be monitored frequently to ensure that ventilator pressures are weaned as compliance improves. Parameters should be established for repeat surfactant dosing and shared with the health care team so the practitioner is notified in a timely fashion of subsequent dosing needs. Blood gas monitoring aids in adjusting or initiating mechanical ventilation. Permissive hypercarbia, keeping carbon dioxide levels upper 40s to 60 mm Hg and pH greater than 7.25, is a general goal.[26] The main priority is to provide only the support needed and to avoid hyperventilation and volutrauma. Environmental and nonpharmacologic comfort measures should be provided during ventilatory support, along with analgesics or sedatives as indicated.

It is important to consider and acquire umbilical lines soon after birth. If the infant is requiring ventilatory assistance, the arterial line can assist with heart rate and blood pressure monitoring, along with arterial blood gas sampling. An umbilical venous catheter or percutaneously inserted central catheter provides central venous access for blood sampling and central parenteral nutrition. Umbilical catheters should be secured, to maintain the line without slipping or loss. A line that slips one half centimeter can mean the difference between a properly placed line and displacement in the ELBW infant. Some practitioners prefer to suture the lines in place and support the suture by applying a tape tab over the suture, securing it to the catheter, instead of securing the line to the abdomen using an adhesive product. One should remove any disinfectant used to clean the cord (chlorhexidine or povidone-iodine) with sterile water or saline to remove any residual product that might cause tissue damage.[27] When central lines are indicated following birth, it is best to avoid any unnecessary skin punctures or peripheral intravenous lines when possible. Skin punctures increase the risk for infection[28] and add stress for the infant.

Blood pressure is a vital sign that should be monitored closely in the ELBW infant. These infants do not have the ability to differentiate cerebral perfusion from systemic perfusion.[17] Therefore, if systemic pressure is inadequate, then cerebral perfusion should be in question. The best continuous method for evaluating the ELBW infant's blood pressure is by way of a functioning arterial line. The mean blood pressure should be at least the infant's gestational age in weeks.[29] Hypotension is common in the ELBW infant and is most commonly due to adrenocortical insufficiency, poor vascular tone, and immature catecholamine response, rather than hypovolemia.[30] Therefore, dopamine and physiologic doses of hydrocortisone are commonly used to treat ELBW hypotension.[31] It is also important to ensure and maintain an adequate hematocrit of 40% to 50%.[32] Perfusion is also essential to evaluate when determining if a blood pressure is adequate. The distal extremity pulses should be palpable and the extremities should have capillary refill less than 2 seconds and should be warm to the touch. Urine output should be at least 0.5 mL/kg/hour on the first day of life and rise to 1 to 2 mL/kg/hour,[33] with a stable bicarbonate level between 19 and 22 mm Hg and an adequate blood pH of 7.25 to 7.35.[18] When tissues are perfused inadequately, the cells will transition to anaerobic metabolism and produce lactic acid, which will drop the body's pH and bicarbonate levels.

The goal of fluid management in the first few days of life should be to replace losses (through skin, urine output, respiration, and so forth). ELBW infants at 23 to 25 weeks' gestation have 10 times higher transepidermal water loss (TEWL) than term infants.[34] Several techniques can be used to minimize TEWL in the ELBW infant. Placing the infant after delivery in an occlusive polyethylene bag up to his/her shoulders until admission into the NICU is a first step.[34] Providing a 70% to 90% relative humidity level is an additional technique that can minimize fluid loss by up to one half in the ELBW population.[35] A preservative-free, water-miscible, petrolatum-based emollient can also be used to keep the skin moist and free from drying, fissures, or flaking. Care should be taken when using these products regularly and frequently during the first couple of weeks of life because an association with coagulase-negative *Staphylococcus epidermidis* infection has been reported.[36]

Phototherapy is almost always required during the first days of the ELBW infant's life. The skin is extremely fragile and bruises during the birth process and the immature liver does not process bilirubin efficiently. At times, practitioners order phototherapy on admission to the NICU knowing that the initial bilirubin level will indicate a need for treatment. Several phototherapy lights minimize TEWL. They include the fluorescent (banklight) and new light-emitting diode (LED) phototherapy lights.[37] Eye shades used during phototherapy can be maintained under a hat without the need to apply adhesive to the skin, which may cause epidermal stripping, and without the need for a circumferential band around the head.

Most health care providers start the ELBW infant at 80 to 120 mL/kg/day of fluid and adjust the amount administered by evaluating electrolyte levels every 6 to 12 hours, body weight every 12 to 24 hours (bed scales are optimal), and urine output over the first couple of days of life. Sodium (133–148 mEq/L) and chloride (100–115 mEq/L) levels[38] are sensitive indicators of fluid levels in the first days of life, especially if minimal sodium has been administered by way of medications or intravenous fluids. Providing only the fluid required to maintain hydration will avoid overload, which should support ductal closure.

When monitoring electrolyte levels, it is also important to assess the glucose level. Ten percent dextrose–containing fluid is usually initiated in the NICU and this dextrose concentration may need to be adjusted down if the glucose level rises higher than 150 mg/dL. Dextrose 4.7% is the lowest glucose concentration that can be administered without electrolytes.[39] When glucose levels reach 250 mg/dL, the infant should be assessed for osmotic diuresis, which results in an increased urine output and could lead to dehydration. Some ELBW infants require supplemental insulin to maintain acceptable glucose levels.

Parenteral nutrition should be initiated as soon as venous access is placed in the ELBW infant. These infants require protein administration of 2 g/kg/day and 50 to 60 kcal/kg/day to avoid a negative nitrogen balance and a catabolic state.[40] Many NICUs prepare a general admission TPN solution with at least dextrose and protein for premature infants born throughout the 24-hour period. Over time, protein should be increased to 2.25 to 4 g/kg/day to support growth.[41] Intralipid 20%, 0.5 g/kg/day, is a parenteral fat solution, that can be initiated on the first or second day of life and titrated up as triglyceride levels indicate tolerance of less than 200 mg/dL.[42] Minimal enteral feeding or trophic feeding (12–24 mL/kg/day)[43] should be considered as soon as the ELBW infant is stable. Breast milk is the preferred substrate.[40] The mother should be encouraged to pump and collect colostrum for her infant's important initial feedings.

It is essential to provide care to the ELBW infant in a supported, quiet, and dim environment. The experienced health care provider can monitor and provide care with minimal handling while supporting longer rest periods. ELBW infants are sensitive to noxious odors.[44] One should take care to minimize the use of cleaning products (alcohol) on, or near, these infants. Perfume, after-shave, clothing exposed to tobacco smoke, and so forth, should be kept away from these infants during their early NICU course.

We need to educate parents on how to maintain the therapeutic environment while interacting with their infant. Placing a parent's palm on the infant's head maybe well tolerated, whereas stroking the infant's foot may not. The parents or family can be encouraged to bring in a dark washcloth or piece of fleece to shield their infant's eyes from bright light. The mother can provide a clean, but worn, breast pad to place near the infant's face to expose the infant to his/her mother's scent.

Parents need to be our partners during the first few days of the ELBW infant's life and throughout the hospitalization. They will need to be educated about their infant's condition and will need to discuss issues that are of concern. The more the parents are involved early in the care, the better prepared they will be to make decisions for their child.

CASE PRESENTATION

AE is a 38year-old, gravida 5, para 0 woman at 23 weeks' gestation who has a history of spontaneous habitual abortions. She presented to a community emergency department with vomiting and diarrhea while on vacation. She was diagnosed with preterm labor, assessed as 3 cm dilated, given steroids, a tocolytic, fluids, and antibiotics, and emergently transported to the regional perinatal center.

On arrival at the perinatal center, she was found to be febrile, with a white blood cell count of 22, and was 6 cm dilated, and labor was progressing rapidly. Because chorioamnionitis was highly suspected, another antibiotic was administered and the team prepared for an ELBW birth. She was seen by a perinatologist and a neonatologist who all agreed to try to resuscitate and stabilize the neonate per the parents' request. This couple had wanted a baby for years and was well educated about the potential complications of delivering their daughter at 23 weeks' gestation.

Baby Girl E was spontaneously vaginally delivered 7 hours after AE's initial presentation at the referring hospital. She was born vigorous, with a weak cry, weighing 525 g. CPAP was applied to assist her work of breathing and to help her maintain a functional residual capacity. On admission to the NICU, her saturations were 93% on 30% F_{IO_2}, with only a mild increased work of breathing. She was well perfused and active. Baby Girl E's extremities were kept flexed, with her body swaddled in a U-shaped boundary and her head and neck maintained in a midline position. Because of her age, the potential for infection, and need for optimal nutritional support, an umbilical venous line was placed. Her initial white blood cell count was three with a marked left shift, and ampicillin and gentamicin were administered. An arterial catheter was also placed to monitor her central blood pressure along with blood gases because she was extremely premature and did not have the advantage of a full course of maternal steroids.

Baby Girl E did extremely well during the first 12 hours of life (referred to as the honeymoon) until she started to have apneic episodes, an increased CO_2 level of 64, decreased pH of 7.20, and an increased work of breathing. Her chest radiograph showed moderate diffuse granularity with air bronchograms, consistent with respiratory distress syndrome. She was intubated, placed on synchronized intermittent mechanical ventilation, and given a dose of surfactant. Over the next 12 hours, she weaned to minimal ventilatory settings. Her parents and grandparents spent a great deal of time at the bedside. They were extremely concerned about her being comfortable and worried about her ultimate prognosis, given mom's probable chorioamnionitis.

On day of life #2, Baby Girl E became poorly perfused and hypotensive. She was acidotic and failing to oxygenate or ventilate. She was switched over to an oscillator in the hopes of optimizing pulmonary function while minimizing barotrauma of her premature lungs. A volume bolus was administered without improving perfusion, so dopamine was initiated, followed by dobutamine and epinephrine. A third antibiotic was initiated because septic shock was highly likely the cause of her deterioration. Over the next 12 hours, she received blood products, hydrocortisone to support her low cortisol level, and maximal inotropic support to try to maintain an adequate cardiac output. In the meantime, she required more ventilatory support, which resulted in a right pneumothorax, requiring a chest tube. In consultation with the parents, the attending neonatologist ordered a neural ultrasound, knowing that this infant was at extreme risk for an IVH because of her age and instability. The neural ultrasound demonstrated a bilateral grade 4 bleed with marked diffuse PVL. As a fetus, Baby Girl E had experienced a prior neural insult in utero, most likely from a thrombus. After consultation with the family and their chaplain, the parents decided to withdraw support and provide comfort care to their gravely ill daughter. While the parents were at her bedside, they spoke fondly of the brief time they had shared with her and the wonderful memories they had. Mom held her daughter as this tiny infant died peacefully surrounded by her family.

SUMMARY

Caring for the ELBW infant in the first days of life is complex and challenging, yet rewarding. We never know what memories or time will be held as most precious by the family. It is the experienced health care provider who will be best prepared to meet the needs of these fragile infants and their concerned/frightened parents. Understanding how to minimize stress and support body functions will enable us to better care for these infants in the first few days of life. We should strive to partner with parents, using respectful communication and encouraging decision making, even in the resuscitative and stabilization phases of care, particularly when an infant may not survive. Nursing plays an essential role in providing this minute-to-minute support. It is not always what we do, but how we do it, that may matter most.

ACKNOWLEDGMENT

Special thanks to Gretchen Lawhon, RN, PhD, NIDCAP Master Trainer, Director, Mid-Atlantic NIDCAP Center, for her thoughtful review and suggestions to enhance this article.

REFERENCES

1. Sutramanian K, Barton A, Montazami S. Extremely low birth weight infant. Available at: www.emedicine.com. Accessed January 6, 2008.
2. American Academy of Pediatrics. Preterm labor. In: Perinatal continuing education program: maternal and fetal care. Elk Grove Village (IL): AAP; 2007. p. 287.
3. American Academy of Pediatrics. Fetal age, growth, and maturity. In: Perinatal continuing education program: maternal and fetal evaluation and immediate newborn care. Elk Grove Village (IL): AAP; 2007. p. 46.
4. American Academy of Pediatrics. Preterm labor. In: Perinatal continuing education program: maternal and fetal care. Elk Grove Village (IL): AAP; 2007. p. 296.
5. Gomella TL, Cunningham MD, Eyal FG, et al. Neurologic diseases. In: Neonatology: management, procedures, on-call problems, diseases, and drugs. New York: Lange Medical Books/McGraw-Hill; 2004. p. 491–2.
6. Gomella TL, Cunningham MD, Eyal FG, et al. Neurologic diseases. In: Neonatology: management, procedures, on-call problems, diseases, and drugs. New York: Lange Medical Books/McGraw-Hill; 2004. p. 493.
7. Gomella TL, Cunningham MD, Eyal FG, et al. Retinopathy of prematurity. In: Neonatology: management, procedures, on-call problems, diseases, and drugs. New York: Lange Medical Books/McGraw-Hill; 2004. p. 559.
8. Askin D, Diehl-Jones W. Ophthalmologic and auditory disorders. In: Verklan MT, Walden M, editors. Core curriculum for neonatal intensive care nursing. St Louis (MO): Elsevier Saunders; 2004. p. 924.
9. Gomella TL, Cunningham MD, Eyal FG, et al. Necrotizing enterocolitis and spontaneous intestinal perforation. In: Neonatology: management, procedures, on-call problems, diseases, and drugs. New York: Lange Medical Books/McGraw-Hill; 2004. p. 483.
10. American Academy of Pediatrics and American College of Obstetricians and Gynecologists. Inpatient perinatal care services. In: Guidelines for perinatal care. Elk Grove Village (IL): AAP; 2007. p. 23–4.
11. American Academy of Pediatrics and American College of Obstetricians and Gynecologists. Interhospital care of the perinatal patient. In: Guidelines for perinatal care. Elk Grove Village (IL): AAP; 2007. p. 67.
12. Karlsen K. Temperature. In: The S.T.A.B.L.E. program: post-resuscitation/pre-transportation stabilization care of sick infants: guidelines for neonatal healthcare providers. Park City (UT): The S.T.A.B.L.E. Program; 2006. p. 51.
13. Kattwinkel J. Resuscitation of babies born premature. In: Neonatal resuscitation textbook. Elk Grove Village (IL): AAP; 2006. p. 8–5.
14. Karlsen K. Temperature. In: The S.T.A.B.L.E. program: post-resuscitation/pre-transportation stabilization care of sick infants: guidelines for neonatal healthcare providers. Park City (UT): The S.T.A.B.L.E. Program; 2006. p. 50.
15. Kattwinkel J. Resuscitation of babies born premature. In: Neonatal resuscitation textbook. Elk Grove Village (IL): AAP; 2006. p. 8–6.
16. Goldberg R, Joshi A, Moscoso P, et al. The effect of head position on intracranial pressure in the neonate. Crit Care Med 1983;11(6):428–30.
17. Gomella TL, Cunningham MD, Eyal FG, et al. Neurologic diseases. In: Neonatology: management, procedures, on-call problems, diseases, and drugs. New York: Lange Medical Books/McGraw-Hill; 2004. p. 492.
18. American Academy of Pediatrics. Review: is the baby sick? Identifying and caring for sick and at-risk infants. In: Perinatal continuing education program: specialized newborn care. Elk Grove Village (IL): AAP; 2007. p. 17.

19. Kendig J, Ryan F, Sinkin R, et al. Comparison of two strategies for surfactant prophylaxis in very premature infants: a muticenter randomized trial. Pediatrics 1998;101(6):1009–11.

20. American Academy of Pediatrics. Surfactant therapy In: Perinatal continuing education program: specialized newborn care. Elk Grove Village (IL): AAP; 2007. p. 172.

21. Turnage-Carrier C, McLane KM, Gregurich MA. Interface pressure comparison of healthy premature infants with various neonatal bed surfaces. Adv Neonatal Care 2008;8(3):178–9.

22. Karlsen K. Temperature. In: The S.T.A.B.L.E. program: post-resuscitation/pre-transportation stabilization care of sick infants: guidelines for neonatal healthcare providers. Park City (UT): The S.T.A.B.L.E. Program; 2006. p. 46.

23. Association of Women's Health, Obstetric and Neonatal Nurses. Adhesives. In: Neonatal skin care: evidence-based clinical practice guide. Washington, DC: AWHONN; 2007. p. 38.

24. Association of Women's Health, Obstetric and Neonatal Nurses. Adhesives. In: Neonatal skin care: evidence-based clinical practice guide. Washington, DC: AWHONN; 2007. p. 37.

25. Maguire DP. Care of the extremely low birth weight infant. In: Verklan MT, Walden M, editors. Core curriculum for neonatal intensive care nursing. St Louis (MO): Elsevier Saunders; 2004. p. 474.

26. American Academy of Pediatrics. Assisted ventilation with mechanical ventilation. In: Perinatal continuing education program: specialized newborn care. Elk Grove Village (IL): AAP; 2007. p. 142.

27. Association of Women's Health, Obstetric and Neonatal Nurses. Disinfectants. In: Neonatal skin care: evidence-based clinical practice guide. Washington, DC: AWHONN; 2007. p. 32.

28. Kilbride H, Powers D, Wirtschafter D, et al. Evaluation and development of potentially better practices to prevent nosocomial bacteremia. Pediatrics 2003; 111(4):e504–18.

29. Carteaux P, Cohen H, Check J, et al. Evaluation and development of potentially better practices for the prevention of brain hemorrhage and ischemic brain injury in very low birth weight infants. Pediatrics 2003;111(4):e489–96.

30. Gomella TL, Cunningham MD, Eyal FG, et al. Hypotension and shock. In: Neonatology: management, procedures, on-call problems, diseases, and drugs. New York: Lange Medical Books/McGraw-Hill; 2004. p. 274.

31. Gomella TL, Cunningham MD, Eyal FG, et al. Hypotension and shock. In: Neonatology: management, procedures, on-call problems, diseases, and drugs. New York: Lange Medical Books/McGraw-Hill; 2004. p. 277.

32. Gomella TL, Cunningham MD, Eyal FG, et al. Hypotension and shock. In: Neonatology: management, procedures, on-call problems, diseases, and drugs. New York: Lange Medical Books/McGraw-Hill; 2004. p. 275.

33. Gomella TL, Cunningham MD, Eyal FG, et al. Management of low weight infant during the first week of life. In: Neonatology: management, procedures, on-call problems, diseases, and drugs. New York: Lange Medical Books/McGraw-Hill; 2004. p. 123.

34. Association of Women's Health, Obstetric and Neonatal Nurses. Transepidermal water loss. In: Neonatal skin care: evidence-based clinical practice guide. Washington, DC: AWHONN; 2007. p. 43.

35. Association of Women's Health, Obstetric and Neonatal Nurses. Transepidermal water loss. In: Neonatal skin care: evidence-based clinical practice guide. Washington, DC: AWHONN; 2007. p. 44.

36. Association of Women's Health, Obstetric and Neonatal Nurses. Emollients. In: Neonatal skin care: evidence-based clinical practice guide. Washington, DC: AWHONN; 2007. p. 41.

37. Association of Women's Health, Obstetric and Neonatal Nurses. Transepidermal water loss. In: Neonatal skin care: evidence-based clinical practice guide. Washington, DC: AWHONN; 2007. p. 45.

38. American Academy of Pediatrics. Review: is the baby sick? Identifying and caring for sick and at-risk infants. In: Perinatal continuing education program: specialized newborn care. Elk Grove Village (IL): AAP; 2007. p. 19.

39. Gomella TL, Cunningham MD, Eyal FG, et al. Hyperglycemia. In: Neonatology: management, procedures, on-call problems, diseases, and drugs. New York: Lange Medical Books/McGraw-Hill; 2004. p. 251.

40. Thureen PJ, Hay WW. Early aggressive nutrition in preterm infants. Semin Neonatol 2001;6:403–15.

41. Gomella TL, Cunningham MD, Eyal FG, et al. Nutritional management. In: Neonatology: management, procedures, on-call problems, diseases, and drugs. New York: Lange Medical Books/McGraw-Hill; 2004. p. 77.

42. Gomella TL, Cunningham MD, Eyal FG, et al. Nutritional management. In: Neonatology: management, procedures, on-call problems, diseases, and drugs. New York: Lange Medical Books/McGraw-Hill; 2004. p. 96.

43. Bakewell-Sachs S, Brandes A. Nutritional management. In: Verklan MT, Walden M, editors. Core curriculum for neonatal intensive care nursing. St Louis (MO): Elsevier Saunders; 2004. p. 224.

44. Liu WF, Laudert S, Perkins B, et al. The development of potentially better practices to support the neurodevelopment of infants in the NICU. J Perinatol 2007;27:s48–74.

Principles of Genetics and Their Clinical Application in the Neonatal Intensive Care Unit

Julieanne H. Schiefelbein, M App Sc, MA(Ed), Cert Hum Gen, NM, NNP-BC, PNP-BC[a,b,c],*, Susan E. Cheeseman, RN, MSN, NNP-BC[d]

KEYWORDS

- Neonatal • Newborn • Genetics • Chromosomes
- Cystic fibrosis • Genetic counseling
- Beckwith-Wiedemann syndrome

The neonate born with a genetic defect or congenital anomaly presents a challenge to the neonatal intensive care unit (NICU) team. A definitive diagnosis is essential for management and care of the neonate and the neonate's family. Genetic disorders or diseases are all congenital, although they may not be expressed or recognized until later in life. Unusual physical features and developmental delay often are later findings that lead to a genetic work-up and possible diagnosis.

Genetic events can result in congenital malformations in early development stages. These congenital malformations are caused by gene mutations or chromosomal structural or numerical anomalies. Genetic diseases may be divided into single-gene defects, multiple-gene disorders, or chromosomal defects. Single-gene defects may arise from abnormalities of both copies of an autosomal gene (a recessive disorder) or of only one of the two copies (a dominant disorder).

Some conditions may result from deletions or abnormalities of a few genes located contiguously on a chromosome. Chromosomal disorders can involve the duplication or loss of larger portions of a chromosome (or an entire chromosome) containing hundreds of genes. Large chromosomal abnormalities affect multiple body parts and different organ systems, whereas smaller ones may be evidenced by a single mild physical feature.

Typically genetic disorders are thought of as being rare; however, this is not true, and it is becoming increasingly evident as knowledge and technology progress. This article includes information on basic genetics, the characteristics and causes of some common congenital malformations, and a systematic process for the evaluation of the malformed infant. Refer to **Table 1** for definitions of common genetic terminology. Commonalities of patient care management issues are addressed, with the understanding that every family requires individualized care. Geneticists and nursing staff also play a key role in assisting families and the medical home in identifying and managing the special health care needs of children who have genetic disorders.

AUTOSOMAL DISORDERS
Autosomal Dominant Disorders

Characteristics of autosomal dominant disorders are that males and females are affected equally and either parent can pass the gene on to sons

[a] Neonatal Nurse Practitioner Service (PCMC), Intermountain Health Care, Salt Lake City, UT, USA
[b] Primary Children's Medical Center, Salt Lake City, UT, USA
[c] College of Nursing, University of Utah, Salt Lake City, UT, USA
[d] Department of Neonatology, St. Luke's Children's Hospital, Boise, ID, USA
* Corresponding author. Neonatal Nurse Practitioner Service (PCMC), Intermountain Health Care, 100 North Mario Capecchi Drive, Salt Lake City, UT 84119.
E-mail address: julieanne.schiefelbein@imail.org (J.H. Schiefelbein).

Crit Care Nurs Clin N Am 21 (2009) 67–85
doi:10.1016/j.ccell.2008.09.005

Table 1
Terminology

Allele	One of a series of alternate forms of a gene at the same location (locus) on a chromosome
Anaphase lag	Chromosome lag during third state of division of a cell nucleus in meiosis and mitosis
Autosomes	The 22 pairs of chromosomes other than the sex-determining chromosomes (the X and Y)
Birth defect	An abnormality of structure, function, or metabolism, whether genetically determined or a result of environmental interference during embryonic or fetal life. A congenital defect may cause disease from the time of conception through birth or later in life.
Chromosome	Structural elements in a cell nucleus that carry the genes and convey genetic information. Each cell (except erythrocytes) in the body contains all the chromosomes received from both parents within its nucleus. There are 23 pairs of chromosomes, for a total of 46 chromosomes, with one maternal and one paternal chromosome creating each pair.
Chromosome lag	Failure of a chromosome to travel to the appropriate daughter cell
Consanguinity	The mating of related individuals
Deletion	Loss of a chromosomal segment
Diploid	Cell containing two copies of each chromosome, a set of maternal and a set of paternal chromosomes, for a total of 46 chromosomes
Dominant gene	A gene that is expressed in the heterozygous state. In a dominant disorder, the mutant gene overshadows the normal gene. A dose of this gene is needed for expression.
Duplication	Any duplication of a region of DNA that contains a gene. It is a process that can result in free mutation.
Environmental influences	Inadequate nutritional intake, certain drugs, irradiation, and viruses are examples that could alter the genetic make-up of an offspring while in vitro.
Gamete	One of two germ cells, containing 23 chromosomes (haploid number)
Gene	The smallest unit of inheritance of a single characteristic, responsible for a physical, biochemical, or physiologic trait and located with other genes in linear sequence along the chromosome.
Genotype	The hereditary composition of an individual; also refers to the specific set of alleles inherited at a locus
Haploid	Refers to cells that have on one copy of each chromosome, characteristic of a gamete (egg or sperm) cell with 23 chromosomes
Heterogenous chromosomes	Differing pair of chromosomes, one from each parent, arraying differing genes for specific traits. When there are unlike genes on a locus, one gene dominates.
Homologous chromosomes	A matched pair of chromosomes, one from each parent, carrying the genes for the same traits
Imprinting	Process in which genetic material is uniquely expressed differently depending on whether inherited from the mother or the father.
Inversion	Occurs when a segment of the chromosome breaks off and reattaches in the reverse direction
Karyotype	Pictorial representation of the chromosomal characteristics of a single cell cut and arranged in pairs based on their size and banding pattern according to a standard classification
Locus	The physical site or location that a gene occupies on a chromosome
Multifactorial	Genes plus environment
Nondisjunction	Failure of paired chromosomes to separate during cell division
Nonmultiples	Designated by the suffix "somy." Monosomy is one less than the diploid number (45) and trisomy is one more than the diploid number (47).

(continued on next page)

Table 1 (continued)	
Nonreciprocal translocation	A one-way transfer of a chromosomal segment to another chromosome
Mosaicism	Nondisjunction of an anaphase lag that occurs during mitosis after fertilization resulting in two different cell lines in the same person
Penetrance	The degree to which an inherited trait is manifested in the person who carries the affected gene
Phenotype	The observable physical and biochemical characteristics of the expression of a gene; the clinical presentation of an individual produced by the interaction of genes and the environment
Polygenic defects	A type of inheritance in which a trait depends on many different gene pairs with cumulative effects
Polyploidy	More than two sets of homologous chromosomes, showing a haploid number
Recessive gene	A gene whose effect is masked or hidden unless both genes of a set of homologous chromosomes at a given locus are abnormal, thus showing the disease. In a heterozygote (carrier) the normal gene overshadows the mutant gene.
Sex chromosomes	The X and Y chromosomes, which are responsible for sex determination—XX for female and XY for male
Translocation	Occurrence of a chromosomal segment at an abnormal site, either on another chromosome or in the wrong position on the same chromosome (eg, an inversion)

or daughters. An affected offspring has an affected parent if the mutation is not new. Half the sons and half the daughters of an affected parent can be anticipated to have the disorder. There is a 50% chance with each pregnancy. Unaffected offspring of an affected parent have all normal offspring if the mate is an unaffected person (assuming complete penetrance).

If two affected people mate, however, three fourths of their offspring will be affected. A double dose of the mutant gene in any of the offspring results in a lethal anomaly (except in the case of Huntington disease). Family history of an anomaly indicates a vertical route of transmission through successive generations on one side of the family (if not a new mutation). Examples of autosomal dominant disorders are myotonic dystrophy, neurofibromatosis, and coronary artery disease[1,2]

Autosomal Recessive Disorders

Males and females are affected equally by autosomal recessive disorders. Parents of affected offspring are rarely affected and are usually heterozygous carriers. After the birth of an affected offspring, there is a 25% chance, with each pregnancy, of having another affected offspring and a 50% chance that the offspring will be a carrier. There may be a distant relative who has the disorder.

Affected people who mate with unaffected people have offspring who are heterozygous carriers. If two affected people mate, all offspring are affected. If there is no family history this indicates a horizontal route of transmission in the same generation. There can be a difference in expression of the disorder from mild in one member to extremely severe in another. Examples of autosomal recessive disorders are cystic fibrosis (CF), sickle cell anemia, Tay-Sachs disease, and thalassemia major.[2,3]

X-LINKED DISORDERS
X-Linked Dominant Disorders

Characteristics of X-linked dominant disorders include that both sexes can be affected; because females have a double chance of receiving the mutant X chromosome, they have twice the risk for being affected. Affected males have all affected daughters and no affected sons. Affected females transmit the disorders in the same manner as with autosomal dominant patterns. Two thirds of the time, affected females have an affected mother; one third of the time, they have an affected father. Family history reveals no father-to-son transmissions. An example is Vitamin D–resistant rickets.[3]

X-Linked Recessive Disorders

One characteristic of X-linked recessive disorders is that only male offspring are affected, with rare exceptions. A female offspring will be affected if she has both a carrier mother and an affected father. Carrier females transmit the disorder. All sons of affected males are normal, whereas all daughters of affected males are carriers (with each pregnancy). Heterozygous females transmit the gene to half their sons, who are affected, and to half their daughters, who are carriers. Transmission is horizontal among males in the same generation; in addition, a generation is skipped, and second-generation males are affected. Examples are Duchenne muscular dystrophy, hemophilia, color blindness, and glucose-6-phosphate dehydrogenase deficiency.[3]

MITOCHONDRIAL DISORDERS

Most genetic diseases are caused by defects in the nuclear genome. A small but significant number of diseases are the result of mitochondrial mutations, however. Because of the unique properties of mitochondria, these diseases display characteristic modes of inheritance and a large degree of phenotypic variability.[4] The mitochondria, which produce adenosine triphosphate (ATP), have their own unique DNA. Mitochondrial DNA is maternally inherited and has a high mutation rate. Organ systems with large ATP requirements and high thresholds tend to be the ones most seriously affected by mitochondrial diseases. For example, the central nervous system consumes 20% of the body's ATP production and is often affected by mtDNA mutations. Mitochondrial mutations are also involved in some common human diseases (eg, a form of deafness).[4]

CHROMOSOMAL DEFECTS

Chromosomal aberrations are disruptions in the normal chromosomal content of a cell and are a major cause of genetic conditions in humans, such as trisomy 21. Chromosomal defects fall into two categories: abnormal number or abnormal structure. Some chromosome abnormalities do not cause disease in carriers, such as translocations or chromosomal inversions. Abnormal numbers of chromosomes or chromosome sets may be lethal or give rise to genetic disorders. Nonmultiples are designated by the suffix "somy": monosomy is one less than the diploid number (45) and trisomy is one more that the diploid (47). The causes of abnormal number include but are not limited to nondisjunction, chromosome lag, anaphase lag, and mosaicism. Abnormalities in chromosome structure follow a chromosome break and the reunion of the wrong segments of the chromosome during the repair process. If, following repair, there is a loss or gain of chromosomal

material (ie, an unbalanced arrangement) there can be significant clinical consequences. If there is no loss or gain of chromosomal material (ie, a balanced rearrangement) then the individual is physically and intellectually normal. There is an increased risk for having chromosomally abnormal offspring, however, because individuals who carry balanced chromosome rearrangements may produce chromosomally unbalanced gametes.

BASIC GENERALIZATIONS

The loss of an entire autosome is usually incompatible with life. One X chromosome is necessary for life and development. If the male-determining Y chromosome is missing, life and development may continue but follows female pathways. Extra entire chromosomes, the translocation of extra chromatin material, and the insertion of extra chromatin material are often compatible with life and development. Multiple congenital structural defects are present when gross aberrations are present.[5]

Incidence

Autosomal aberrations: 1:200 births
Sex chromosome aberrations: 1:500 births
Spontaneous abortions: 60% are associated with chromosomal aberration.[4]

SYSTEMATIC APPROACH TO EVALUATION OF AN INFANT WHO HAS A GENETIC CONDITION

Complete diagnosis is the essential part of planning care and prognosis. Consideration of the infant's overall problems, in addition to the malformation, is essential.

Evaluation of an Infant who has a Congenital Malformation

A congenital malformation is a structural or functional abnormality of the body that is present from birth. The effects of a birth defect may be either immediate or delayed until later in life. Refer to **Table 2** for an overview of a physical examination.

An infant's history falls into three categories, family history, prenatal history, and neonatal history. A complete family history must include three generations and details of defects in the family history related to the problem in the neonate. It must review and compare medical records or photos of similarly affected relatives. Any history of consanguinity must be noted. A thorough review of reproductive history must be taken, including such occurrences as frequent spontaneous abortions or neonatal or

Table 2
Physical examination

General	Asymmetry, problems of relationship, inappropriate size and strength
Face	Configuration; centered features with normal spacing; round, triangular, flat, birdlike, elfin, coarse, or expressionless characteristics
Head	Size of anterior fontanelle, prominence of frontal bone, flattened or prominent occiput, abnormalities in shape (proportionally large or small)
Skin	Intact, or presence of skin tags, open sinuses, tracts
Hair	Texture, hairline, presence of whorls
Eyes	Structure and color of iris, presence of colobomas, centering and spacing of epicanthal folds (hypotelorism or hypertelorism), ptosis, slanting, eyelash length
Ears	Protruding or prominent shape, location, low set, unilateral or bilateral defect, presence and degree of rotation
Nose	Beaked, bulbous, pinched, upturned, misshapen, two nares, flattened bridge, patency, centered on face
Oral	Intact palate, presence of smooth philtrum, natal teeth; shape and size of tongue, mouth, jaw (micrognathia)
Neck	Short or webbed, redundant folds
Chest	Symmetric; presence of accessory nipples
Abdomen	Number of cord vessels, presence of abdominal wall defects and abdominal musculature, prune belly
Genitourinary system (male)	Hypospadias—four degrees, dependent on placement of meatus; chordee; ambiguous genitalia; testes descended
Anus	Position, patency
Spine	Intact, scoliosis, lordosis, kyphosis
Extremities	Length, shape, absence of bones
Hands and feet	Broad, square, or spadelike shape, polydactyly, clinodactyly, syndactyly, abnormal creases in the palm of the hand (simian or Sydney creases), contractures, abnormally large or small size, overriding fingers, proximally placed thumb, rocker-bottom feet

sudden deaths. The aim of this part of the history is to outline the pattern of inheritance of any identified problems.

A prenatal history must be obtained and includes the number and lengths of all gestations; fetal activity level should also be noted. Maternal exposures to infections, illness, high fevers, medications, radiographic examinations, and known teratogens, such as alcohol, smoking, and use of street and prescription drugs, must all be investigated and recorded. It is also important to review the obstetric factors that may have influence on outcome; these include uterine malformations, complications of labor, and the presenting fetal part.

Important information for diagnosis is often contained within the neonatal history, which includes information such as Apgar scores and growth parameters along with a detailed account of the initial neonatal course, including postnatal events and any specifics of the physical examination and laboratory findings that may have influence on ultimate diagnosis.

GENETIC COUNSELING

Genetic counseling is a communication process that deals with the human problems associated with the occurrence, or the risk for occurrence, of genetic disorders in a family. This process involves collaboration of people from multiple disciplines (physician, sonographer, nurse, genetic counselor, social worker, neonatologist, and pediatric specialist, as indicated) and family support. Genetic counselors provide supportive counseling to families, serve as patient advocates, and refer individuals and families to community or state support services. They serve as educators and resource people for other health care professionals and for the general public.

The principles of genetic counseling are based on correct diagnosis and the pattern of inheritance. It is nondirective in nature, with an emphasis on reinforcement of information previously presented. It is linked to communication with the primary care physician. The goal of genetic counseling is to assist the family in comprehending the diagnostic workup and ultimate diagnosis, role of heredity, recurrence risks and options, possible courses of action, and methods of ongoing adjustment. Firmly grounded in this role are the principles of grief counseling and bereavement support.

Indications for genetic counseling include a previously affected child, parent, or grandparent who has a known or suspected congenital malformation, sensory defect, metabolic disorder, mental retardation, neuromuscular disorder, or degenerative central nervous system disease.[5] Indications also include previously affected cousins who had muscular dystrophy, hemophilia, or hydrocephalus. In addition, any family with a history of consanguinity or recurrent miscarriages should be offered genetic counseling. Those who have had exposure to the hazards of ionizing radiation or concern for teratogenic effects should also be offered genetic services, in addition to women of advanced maternal age or any pregnant woman who has abnormal prenatal test results.

Information is gathered by the following methods: questionnaire, constructing a pedigree, medical records, physical examination, laboratory tests, and carrier detection. A geneticist and genetic counselor provide the family with medical facts, including the differential diagnosis, the risks to fetus and mother, the recommended management for the prenatal course, the type and timing of delivery, and the probable course of the disorder. The long-term care requirements of the infant are also included a thorough explanation of hereditary factors that contribute to the disorder is also addressed.

Many options are available to individuals and couples at risk for a genetic disease in the family, including but not limited to carrier screening, home care of newborn infant, adoption, the appropriate method of termination for gestational age, egg or sperm donation, and prenatal testing. Also included is objective information regarding fetus/neonatal status. At this point statistical risk factors are provided as they relate to this individual fetus. Normal characteristics that can exist in the affected fetus are identified. These are pointed out in pictures to promote awareness of total condition of the fetus.

Assistance is given to families in understanding the causes, risks for recurrence, and the limits of current treatments; this is combined with the discussion of options available for dealing with risk for recurrence. Each option has risks, benefits, and limitations that patients need to understand to choose the option appropriate for them. Much of the information communicated to families can be confusing. Assistance with decision making requires depth in counseling skills and a nondirective approach that is respectful of patient feelings and beliefs. Written information for parents and information regarding support groups is also shared with the family.[2,5,6]

PRENATAL DIAGNOSIS

Recent technology advances and marked progress in the understanding of the etiology and pathogenesis of many common disorders have afforded many families a prenatal diagnosis. Prenatal diagnosis encompasses a range of techniques to determine the health and condition of an unborn fetus. Without knowledge gained by prenatal diagnosis, there could be an untoward outcome for the fetus or the mother or both. Congenital anomalies account for 20% to 25% of all perinatal deaths.[2,7] Refer to **Box 1** for indications for prenatal testing.

ADVANTAGES IN PRENATAL TESTING AND DIAGNOSIS

Through prenatal testing, the family can learn that the fetus is unaffected. If this is not the case the family is given time to explore options and prepare for an affected newborn infant. The opportunity to electively choose either to avoid starting a pregnancy or to abort an affected fetus is also provided by prenatal testing. This knowledge also affords the opportunity for the physician to plan delivery, management, and care of the infant when the disease is diagnosed in the fetus.[4]

There is an array of noninvasive and invasive techniques available for prenatal diagnosis. Each

---

Box 1
Indications for prenatal testing

Advanced maternal age

Previous child with a chromosomal disorder

Family history of neural tube defects

Previous child with multiple malformations

Carriers of chromosome translocations

Couples at risk for having a child with a specific inborn error of metabolism (previous child or by carrier testing)

Ultrasonographic identification of major malformation, polyhydramnios, or intrauterine growth restriction of them can be applied only during specific time periods during the pregnancy for greatest usefulness. Refer to **Box 2** for a list of prenatal tests available.

ULTRASONOGRAPHY

Ultrasonography is a noninvasive procedure that is risk-free to the fetus and the mother. High-frequency sound waves are used to produce visible images from the pattern of the echoes made by different tissues and organs, including the baby in the amniotic cavity. The developing embryo can first be visualized at about 6 weeks' gestation. Recognition of the major internal organs and extremities to determine if any are uncharacteristic can best be accomplished between 16 and 20 weeks' gestation.

Although an ultrasound examination is useful to determine the size and position of the fetus and placenta, the volume of amniotic fluid, the appearance of fetal anatomy, and the verification of gestational age, there are limitations to this procedure. There are subtle abnormalities that may not be detected until later in pregnancy, or may not be detected at all. A common example of this is Down syndrome (trisomy 21) wherein the morphologic abnormalities are often not distinct but appear only as subtle findings, such as nuchal thickening. Other anomalies that can be detected include many that indicate various syndromes. Examples of theses are anencephaly, atrial septal defect, cardiac anomalies, choroid plexus cyst, cleft lip, craniosynostosis, cystic hygroma, cystic kidneys, encephalocele, gastroschisis, hydrocephalus, microcephaly, myelomeningocele, omphalocele, and skeletal dysplasia.[4,5]

AMNIOCENTESIS

An amniocentesis is preceded by an ultrasound to determine the position of the fetus and placenta and confirm that sufficient amniotic fluid is present. Sufficient volume of amniotic fluid is normally present after 14 weeks' gestation. For prenatal diagnosis, most amniocenteses are performed between 14 and 20 weeks' gestation. Amniocentesis is an invasive procedure; with the use of ultrasound guidance a needle is passed through the mother's lower abdomen into the amniotic cavity inside the uterus to obtain amniotic fluid. Contained in the amniotic fluid are fetal cells, which are then grown in culture for chromosome analysis, biochemical analysis, and molecular biologic analysis.

During the third trimester of pregnancy, the amniotic fluid can also be analyzed for determination of fetal lung maturity. The amniotic fluid is analyzed by fluorescence polarization (fpol), for lecithin: sphingomyelin (LS) ratio or for phosphatidyl glycerol (PG). This information is used in determining whether early delivery of the fetus is feasible.

Risks with amniocentesis are infrequent; however, fetal loss and maternal Rh sensitization can occur. The increased risk for fetal mortality following amniocentesis is about 0.5% greater than what would normally be expected. Rh-negative mothers can be treated with RhoGAM. Contamination of fluid from amniocentesis by maternal cells is highly unlikely. If oligohydramnios is present, amniotic fluid cannot routinely be obtained. With the use of amnioinfusion, in which a saline solution is instilled into the amniotic cavity, fluid for analysis can be obtained.

Fluid analysis requires 2 to 3 weeks for cells to grow adequately for accurate analysis. The following information can then be obtained:

Fetal sex: determined through special staining techniques, karyotype, or amniotic fluid testosterone levels, providing risk information for X-linked disorder.

α_1-fetoprotein (AFP): abnormally high or low levels raise concern.

Biochemical: metabolism disorders, including Tay-Sachs disease (a lipid disorder) and amino acid, carbohydrate, and mucopolysaccharide metabolism disorders, can be discovered by 20 weeks' gestation.

Chromosomes: abnormalities, including Down syndrome, other trisomies, and other chromosomal abnormalities, can be detected at 16 weeks' gestation by karyotyping.

During the third trimester of pregnancy, the amniotic fluid can also be analyzed for determination of fetal lung maturity. The amniotic fluid is analyzed by fpol for LS ratio or for PG. This information is used in determining whether early delivery of the fetus is feasible.

CHORIONIC VILLUS SAMPLING

During chorionic villus sampling (CVS), while under ultrasound guidance, a catheter is passed by way

---

Box 2
Techniques used in prenatal diagnosis
Ultrasonography
Amniocentesis
Chorionic villus sampling
Fetal blood cells in maternal blood
Percutaneous umbilical blood sampling
Maternal serum testing (triple and quad screening)

of the vagina through the cervix and uterus (alternative approach is transabdominal) into the developing placenta allowing sampling of cells from the placental chorionic villi. These cells can then be analyzed by various techniques, the most frequent being chromosome analysis. The cells can also be grown in culture for biochemical or molecular biologic analysis. CVS can be safely performed between 9.5 and 12.5 weeks' gestation.

CVS has the drawback of being an invasive procedure, and it has a small but significant rate of morbidity for the fetus; this loss rate is about 0.5% to 1% higher than for women undergoing amniocentesis. Rarely, CVS can be associated with limb defects in the fetus. The possibility of maternal Rh sensitization is present. The possibility that maternal blood cells in the developing placenta will be sampled instead of fetal cells and confound chromosome analysis also exists.

MATERNAL BLOOD SAMPLING FOR FETAL BLOOD CELLS

Maternal blood sampling for fetal blood cells is a fresh technique that makes use of the phenomenon of fetal blood cells gaining access to maternal circulation through the placental villi. Typically, only a minute number of fetal cells enter the maternal circulation in this way (not enough to produce a positive Kleihauer-Betke test for fetal-maternal hemorrhage). The fetal cells can be arranged and analyzed by various techniques looking for exact DNA sequences, but without the risks that these latter two invasive procedures inherently have. Fluorescence in situ hybridization (FISH) is one technique that can be applied to recognize particular chromosomes of the fetal cells recovered from maternal blood and diagnose aneuploid conditions, such as the trisomies and monosomy X. The complexity with this technique is that it is difficult to get sufficient fetal blood cells to reliably determine anomalies of the fetal karyotype or assay for other abnormalities. Contraindications to CVS include multiple gestation, uterine bleeding during the pregnancy, active genital herpes infection or other cervical infection, and uterine fibroids. CVS cannot identify neural tube defects. Fetal cell analysis requires 24 to 48 hours for initial results.

PERCUTANEOUS UMBILICAL BLOOD SAMPLING

Percutaneous umbilical blood sampling (PUBS) is a diagnostic test that examines blood from the fetus to detect fetal abnormalities. Under ultrasound guidance a thin needle is inserted into the umbilical cord to retrieve a small sample of fetal blood. The procedure is similar to amniocentesis except the object is to retrieve blood from the fetus versus obtaining amniotic fluid. The results are typically available within 72 hours. This test can be performed from 18 weeks to term. PUBS is indicated when early test results are desired, such as when an abnormality is identified by ultrasonography late in pregnancy, or when a client has been exposed to infectious disease that could affect development of fetus. PUBS is also useful when there is a suspected diagnosis of blood incompatibility (Rh disease) and if there is a drug or chemical level in fetal blood that needs to be assessed. The risks are the same as amniocentesis and also include perforation of uterine arteries and clotting in the fetal cord. There is a chance of premature delivery. Miscarriage is the primary risk related to cordocentesis, occurring in 1 to 2 out of every 100 procedures.[8]

MATERNAL SERUM TESTING: TRIPLE AND QUAD SCREEN TESTS

Maternal serum testing is a screening test performed at 15 to 20 weeks. The triple screen is a group of three tests that are used to screen pregnant woman in the second trimester of pregnancy. The quad screen adds a fourth test to the group. The test helps evaluate the risk that a fetus has certain abnormalities, including trisomy 21, and neural tube defects. Each test performed measures a different substance found in the blood: AFP, human chorionic gonadotropin (hcG), unconjugated estriol (uE3), and with the quad screen, inhibin A. The newest marker, inhibin A, increases the sensitivity and specificity of the screen. These tests have been established as a triple or quad screen because the power lies in their use together. A mathematical calculation involving the levels of these three or four substances and considerations of maternal age, weight, race, and diabetic status are used to determine a numeric risk for trisomy 21 and other selected chromosomal anomalies (ie, trisomy 18). This risk is compared with an established cutoff. If the risk is higher than the cutoff value, then it is considered positive or increased. In preparation the client is counseled that this is a screening test, not a diagnostic test. It is also explained that an abnormal result does not indicate an abnormality but indicates the possible need for a diagnostic test to rule out an abnormality.

Substances Measured in Maternal Serum Testing

Alpha-fetoprotein (AFP) is a protein produced by fetal tissue. During development, AFP levels in fetal blood and amniotic fluid increase until about 12 weeks; then levels gradually decrease until birth. Some AFP crosses the placenta and appears in the maternal blood.

Human chorionic gonadotropin (hcG) is a hormone produced by the placenta. Levels of hcG increase in maternal blood for the first trimester of pregnancy and then decrease to less than 10% by the end of pregnancy.

Unconjugated estriol (uE3) is a form of estrogen that is produced by the fetus through metabolism. This process involves the liver, adrenals, and placenta. Some of the unconjugated estriol crosses the placenta and can be measured in the mother's blood. Levels increase around the eighth week and continue to increase until shortly before delivery.

Inhibin A is a hormone also produced by the placenta. Inhibin is a dimer (has two parts) and is sometimes referred to as DIA or dimeric inhibin A. Levels in maternal blood decrease slightly from 14 to 17 weeks of gestation and then increase again. Inhibin is secreted by the placenta and the corpus luteum. An increased level of inhibin-A is associated with an increased risk for trisomy. A high inhibin-A may also be associated with a risk for preterm delivery.

Limitations

The test result depends on accurate determination of the gestational age of the fetus. If the gestational age of the fetus has not been accurately determined, the results may be falsely high or low. In multiple-gestation pregnancies calculation of the risk for trisomy 21 or trisomy 18 is difficult. For twin pregnancies, a "pseudorisk" can be calculated comparing results to normal results in other twin pregnancies. For higher-gestation pregnancies, risk cannot be calculated from these tests. The evaluation of the risk for open neural tube defects in twin pregnancies can be determined, although it is not as effective as in singleton pregnancies.

RESULTS AND FURTHER TESTING

A multiple marker test or triple screen is used to determine if a fetus is at an increased risk for having certain congenital abnormalities. The test has a high rate of false positives; as few as 10% of women who have abnormal results go on to have babies who have congenital defects. The purpose of the test is to determine if further testing (such as ultrasound or amniocentesis) is warranted.

POSTNATAL TESTING

Chromosome analysis/karyotype is an ordered display of an individual's chromosomes. This test can be done on amniotic fluid prenatally. Chromosomes are analyzed by staining techniques that result in visibility of dark and light bands that are designated in a standardized way from the centromere during metaphase.

High-resolution banding/prometaphase banding. Some disorders cannot be seen reliably on standard chromosome analysis and require special handling during processing. Prometaphase banding is used because the cell growth during culturing is adjusted to maximize the number of cells in prometaphase, when the chromosomes are much less condensed and therefore longer, rather than in metaphase, when the cell growth is stopped in standard chromosome studies. High-resolution banding can have from 550 to 800 bands and allows a much more detailed analysis.

FISH is a relatively new technique called molecular cytogenetics that combines chromosome analysis with the use of fluorescence-tagged molecular markers (probes) that are applied after the chromosome preparation is produced. This method relies on the phenomenon of hybridization of complementary pieces of DNA. FISH is a powerful tool useful not only in diagnosing relatively common microdeletion or microduplication disorders but also for identifying the origin of extra chromosome material.[1]

Polymerase chain reaction (PCR) is a powerful technique in amplifying many copies of a segment of DNA so that it can be analyzed. PCR is useful in disorders with recurring mutation, such as achondroplasia.

Comparative Genomic Hybridization (CGH) microarray testing. This testing is an advancement in cytogenetic technology that allows detection of cytogenetic imbalances that are smaller than what can be detected through routine chromosome analysis. Testing detects the loss (deletion) or gain (duplication) of chromosomal regions.

Methylation studies evaluate the methylation status of a gene (attachment of methyl groups to DNA cytosine bases); genes that are methylated are not expressed but potentials can be. Methylation pays a role in X-chromosome inactivation and imprinting. Methylation analysis may be used as a diagnostic test in disorders associated with imprinting, including Prader-Willi syndrome, Angelman syndrome, and Beckwith-Wiedemann syndrome (BWS).

COMMON TRISOMY DISORDERS

The vast field of genetic concepts and testing is applicable in a practical way in the recognition and care of patients who have autosomal trisomies.

Trisomy 21 (Down Syndrome)

As illustrated in **Table 3** the risk for trisomy 21 increases with maternal age, with rapid acceleration of risk beyond 35 years of age. Trisomy 21 accounts for 15% to 20% of cases of severe mental retardation. A person who has this trisomy has 47 chromosomes (3 of chromosome 21). The extra chromosome in trisomy 21 is received from the father in 25% of cases. The extra chromosome results from nondisjunction during meiosis, which may occur unrelated to maternal cause and appears as follows:

Chromosomes: 46
Translocation of chromosome 21.
Familial transmission autosomal dominant.
No abnormalities if chromosomes are balanced. There is one No. 21 and one No. 14 chromosome.
Production of unbalanced gametes by balanced carriers: should consider prenatal diagnosis

Some infants have mosaicism for trisomy 21 or translocation 14/21 or 21/22. People who have this mosaicism can have all the defects, whereas others have only a few. It is possible for some of this group to have normal intellectual ability. Refer to **Table 4** for a comparison of the clinical presentation of the three most common trisomies.

Table 3 Risk for trisomy 21 based on maternal age	
Maternal Age (y)	**Incidence**
15–29	1:1500
30–34	1:800
35–39	1:270
40–44	1:100
45 and older	1:50

Many people who have trisomy 21 live productive and normal lives. Complications can occur, however, and these are multiple. About 40% to 50% of infants have heart defects. Some defects are minor and may be treated with medications, whereas others may require surgery. About 10% of infants who have trisomy 21 are born with intestinal malformations that require surgery. Children are at increased risk for visual or hearing impairment also. Upper respiratory tract infections are common in this group. The degree of mental retardation that accompanies trisomy 21 varies widely, ranging from mild to moderate to severe. Most mental retardation falls within the mild to moderate range. There is no way to predict the mental development of a child who has trisomy 21 based on physical features or initial neurologic examination. It is essential that children who have trisomy 21 be referred for early intervention programs beginning in infancy, which allow them to attain their greatest potential.

Trisomy 18 (Edwards Syndrome)

Trisomy 18 is the second most common autosomal trisomy. It is a rare genetic chromosomal syndrome in which the child has an extra or third copy of chromosome 18. The rate of occurrence for trisomy 18 is approximately 1 in 3000 (for conception) and approximately 1 in 5000 to 6000 (for live births), because 50% of those diagnosed prenatally with the condition do not survive the prenatal period. It is much more common at conception, however, and is the most common chromosomal abnormality among stillbirths. Approximately 80% of newborns affected by this disorder are female.

Recent studies indicate a mortality rate of 50% for children who have trisomy 18. Infants normally die within the first 1 to 2 months of life, usually as a result of heart failure.[4] The survival rate decreases to 10% in the first year, and these survivors have severe mental retardation. Many factors contribute to and account for this high rate of mortality; these include aspiration pneumonia, susceptibility to infections, and the sequela of congenital heart defects. Refer to **Table 4** for presenting features and complications associated with trisomy 18.

There is no cure for trisomy 18 and considering that infants have major physical abnormalities, health care providers and parents face difficult choices regarding treatment. Abnormalities can be treated to a certain degree with surgery, but extreme invasive procedures may not be in the best interest of an infant whose life span is measured in days or weeks. Medical therapy often consists of

Table 4
Trisomy 21, 18, and 13

Clinical Presentation	Trisomy 21 (Down Syndrome)	Trisomy 18 (Edwards Syndrome)	Trisomy 13 (Patau Syndrome)
General	Low birth weight, hypotonia	Low birth weight, small for gestational age, hypertonia	Low birth weight, hypotonia
Head	Skull short and round with flat occiput. Flat facies. Cheeks are round, red.	Abnormally prominent occiput. Frontal bossing	Cutis aplasia (scalp defect on the posterior occiput). Cutis hemangiomas.
Eyes	Upslanting short palpebral fissures, prominent epicanthal folds, Brushfield spots: iris may be speckled with a ring of round, grayish spots or flecks of gold in light-colored eyes.	Ptosis (droopiness) of one or both eyelids.	Microphthalmia (small, abnormally formed eyes), colobomas of iris, cataracts.
Mouth and nose	Tongue protrudes, corners of the mouth are sometimes downturned.	Micrognathia (small jaw) and microstomia (small mouth), which may be difficult to open	Oral facial clefts (not always). Broad and flattened nasal bridge.
Ears	Small and sometimes overfolded	Small with unraveled helices	Malformed and low-set
Neck	Short with redundant skin folds	Redundant skin folds	Short with redundant skin folds
Chest	—	Short sternum	—
Skeletal	Narrow acetabular angle. Narrow iliac index. Broadened iliac bones. (On radiograph)	Small pelvis	Hypoplasia of hip
Hands and feet	Broad and short, deep flexion creases across the palms (simian crease) in 50% of infants. Wide space between great toe and second toe	Overlapping fingers with clenched fists, flexion contraction of the two middle digits and unfolded thumbs. Syndactyly. Simian crease (25%). Rocker bottom feet, short big toes	Flexion deformities of hands, fingers and wrists: postaxial polydactyly. Rocker bottom feet.
Additional defects	Structural heart defects in 50% of infants: most common atrioventricular canal and ventricular septal defects (VSDs). Duodenal, esophageal, or anal atresia or stenosis. Leukemia. Conductive and neural hearing loss. Hypothyroidism. Visual disturbances.	Structural heart defects, VSDs most common. Omphalocele, diaphragmatic hernia, occasionally spina bifida.	Structural heart defects, patent ductus arteriosus, or rotational anomalies, such as dextroposition. Gross brain defects, grand mal seizures, myoclonic jerks. Hematologic abnormalities.
Disabilities appearing later	Moderate to severe mental retardation (IQ ranging from 25 to 60)	50% die within the first weeks of life, 95% by the first year of life; marked disabilities	50% die within the first weeks of life, 95% by the first year of life; marked disabilities

supportive care with the goal of making the infant comfortable, rather than prolonging life. This may include gavage or gastric tube feedings as needed for poor oral intake and to sustain nutrition. Oxygen may be needed for respiratory distress. The most crucial form of support for these infants is parental and family support.

Trisomy 13 (Patau Syndrome)

Trisomy 13, also known as Patau Syndrome, may be related to older maternal age. The incidence is 1 in 5000 births. It is a chromosomal abnormality, a syndrome in which a patient has an additional chromosome 13 due to a nondisjunction of chromosomes during meiosis. The extra chromosome 13 disrupts the normal course of development, causing the characteristic features of Patau syndrome or trisomy 13. Like all nondisjunction diseases (trisomy 21 and 18), the risk for disease in the offspring increases with maternal age at pregnancy.

The mortality rate in this group is 44% and most infants die within the first month; survival is 18% at 1 year of life. These infants have severe mental retardation. Refer to **Table 3** for presentation and complications.

Some infants born with trisomy 13 have severe and incurable birth defects. Children who have better prognoses require medical treatment to correct structural abnormalities and associated complications. For feeding problems, special formulas, positions, and techniques may be used. Tube feeding or the placement of a gastrostomy tube may be required. Structural abnormalities, such as cleft lip and cleft palate, can be corrected through surgery. Special diets, hearing aids, and vision aids can be used to mitigate the symptoms of trisomy 13. Physical therapy, speech therapy, and other types of developmental therapy help the child reach his or her potential. Because the translocation form of trisomy 13 is genetically transmitted, genetic counseling for the parents should be part of the management of the disease.

Having an infant who has complex medical problems is stressful for families, who require teaching and emotional support. An important task for the nurses who work with these families in crisis is support, with caring and with the difficult decisions that often arise. If the family desires, social work and chaplaincy support should be offered.

The above-described trisomies are the most common seen in neonatal care. Not all chromosomal anomalies or congenital malformations are diagnosed prenatally. The clinician is then presented with an unusual infant. The following two case studies incorporate the aspects of diagnosis, care management, and options for the patient and family.

CASE REPORT ONE

A female infant, who had prenatally diagnosed omphalocele, was delivered vaginally to a 38-year-old gravida 3 para 1 at 33 weeks and 3 days following premature rupture of membranes for 38 hours. The infant was conceived by in vitro fertilization; prenatal genetics was involved and preconception and prenatal vitamins were taken. Maternal history included two prior pregnancy losses, advanced maternal age, and history of herpes simplex virus with last outbreak 1 year before delivery. Mother's group B streptococcus status was unknown at the time of delivery and remaining prenatal laboratory studies were normal. Intrapartum Unasyn was given because of prolonged rupture of membranes, along with group B streptococcal prophylaxis and betamethasone for fetal surfactant induction. With increased uterine contractions and cervical changes labor was augmented and intrapartum epidural was placed.

The infant presented with respiratory distress, grunting and retracting with diminished breath sounds bilaterally; the physical examination was significant for visible herniated bowel within intact umbilical stalk. Birth weight was 2.1 kg, length 43 cm, and head circumference 30 cm, all appropriate for gestational age. Apgar scores of 8 at 1 minute and 9 at 10 minutes were assigned. The small abdominal wall defect was wrapped in moist sterile gauze before transfer to the NICU.

The infant was intubated and given surfactant. Chest radiograph was consistent with respiratory distress syndrome (RDS). Subsequent physical examination revealed macroglossia and linear creases in the earlobes bilaterally. Routine admission screening showed serum glucose of 29 before initiation of intravenous glucose administration. She required two D10W boluses (2 mg/kg) in addition to intravenous fluid administration of D10W at 80 mL/kg to attain normoglycemia. Echocardiogram soon after admission showed normal anatomy and function with atrial shunt and patent ductus arteriosus. Primary repair of the omphalocele and appendectomy were performed on the day of birth.

The infant's postoperative course was complicated by RDS requiring additional surfactant, and mild hyperbilirubinemia. She was extubated and weaned to room air by day of life seven. Sepsis evaluation initiated on admission was negative. She experienced difficulty advancing to full-volume feeds because of residuals. An upper gastrointestinal evaluation revealed slow transit time in the small bowel and no malrotation. She improved with the addition of ranitidine and reglan. She was noted to again experience mild hypoglycemia when weaning from intravenous glucose administration, which improved without further intervention.

In consultation with the geneticist, work-up for the infant's omphalocele, macroglossia, and linear indentations of earlobe included chromosome analysis and methylation analysis for BWS syndrome. Chromosome analysis revealed normal karyotype, 46, XX. Methylation studies showed hypomethylation of the differentially methylated region (DMR) 2 imprinting center on chromosome 11p15, which is consistent with BWS.

Discussion

BWS is a rare genetic condition that affects growth occurring in 1 in 14,000 births. The incidence may be higher because some infants could possibly go undiagnosed. It occurs in males and females of all ethnic backgrounds. It causes rapid, uneven growth.

Prenatal and perinatal findings include polyhydramnios, premature birth, and fetal macrosomia (large body size).[9] Other features include a long umbilical cord and an enlarged placenta, averaging almost twice the normal weight for gestational age.[10]

Infants who have BWS generally have macroglossia (enlarged tongue) and macrosomia present at birth (birth weight >97th percentile). The characteristic facies of the infant who has BWS include midfacial hypoplasia, prominent eyes with intraorbital creases, prominent occiput, large fontanels, and capillary nevus flammeus on the central forehead and eyelids. Cleft palate has been reported but only rarely.

Structural anomalies associated with BWS include abdominal wall defects, including omphalocele,[10,11] umbilical hernia, and diastasis recti. At birth infants may have characteristic linear indentations of the lobe and peculiar posterior helical ear pits.[12,13] Hemihyperplasia, described as asymmetric overgrowth of a region or regions of the body, can be present at birth or become more evident with growth. Hemihyperplasia may affect segmental regions of the body or selected organs and tissues. Hemihyperplasia involving the face accounts for the enlarged tongue. Visceromegaly involving one or more intra-abdominal organs, including liver, spleen, kidneys, adrenal glands, and pancreas, has been reported in infants who have BWS. Hemihyperplasia may be limited to one side of the body (ipsilateral) or involve opposite sides of the body (contralateral).[7,14]

Neonatal hypoglycemia is well documented (30%–50% of infants).[15] Most cases of hypoglycemia are mild and transient[9]; however, in more severe cases hypoglycemia can persist. If not detected or not treated appropriately, hypoglycemia can pose a significant risk for developmental sequelae. Delayed onset of hypoglycemia, in the first month of life, is occasionally observed.

Hypercalciuria can be found in children who have BWS even in the absence of renal abnormalities as detected on ultrasound examination (22% in BWS as compared with 7%–10% in the general population).[16] This may reflect an underlying primary structural abnormality in the kidneys. Renal anomalies can include medullary dysplasia, duplicated collecting system, nephrocalcinosis, medullary sponge kidney, cystic changes, diverticula, and nephromegaly.[17,18]

Children who have BWS have an increased risk for developing neoplasia, particularly Wilms tumor and hepatoblastoma, but also neuroblastoma, adrenocortical carcinoma, and rhabdomyosarcoma. In addition a wide variety of other tumors, both malignant and benign, have been seen. Estimated risk for tumor development in children who have BWS is 1 in 10. Wilms tumor is the most common cancer in children who have BWS, occurring in about 5% to 7% of all children who have BWS. Most children develop Wilms tumor before their fourth birthday; however children who have BWS can develop Wilms tumor up to 7 or 8 years of age. By 8 years of age 95% of all Wilms tumors have occurred.[19] The second most common cancer in children who have BWS is hepatoblastoma.

Children who have BWS do not usually have mental retardation.[20] Most children who have BWS have normal development if there is no chromosome abnormality[21,22] or medical complications from prematurity, hypoxia, or untreated hypoglycemia.

Although children who have BWS show rapid growth during early childhood, length generally parallels the normal curve at or above the 95th percentile. Growth usually begins to slow after 8 years of age, whereas mean weight remains between 75th and 95th percentile. Advanced bone age based on radiologic findings is more pronounced during the first 4 years and rarely persists into adulthood. After adulthood, complications for individuals who have BWS are infrequent and prognosis is favorable.

The neonatal team responsible for attending high-risk deliveries may be the first to encounter the infant who has BWS. Any one of the prenatal complications associated with BWS may necessitate attendance by the neonatal team at delivery: polyhydramnios, prematurity, macrosomia, or omphalocele. Initial management by the neonatal team involves careful assessment and prompt intervention as indicated.

Initial and ongoing assessment for airway compromise related to macroglossia is indicated. Airway management may be difficult because of the infant's enlarged tongue, making endotracheal intubation challenging.[10]

For the infant who has omphalocele, the initial goal of management is to prevent hypothermia, maintain a sterile environment, and maintain perfusion to bowel. Consult pediatric surgery for surgical abdominal wall repair and postoperative management. If a cardiac anomaly is suspected, a comprehensive cardiac evaluation, including ECG and echocardiogram, needs to be obtained before surgery. If transfer to a tertiary care center is needed, special consideration should be given to maintaining airway and euglycemia with intravenous dextrose.

Evaluation for hypoglycemia and prompt treatment are extremely important in preventing serious compromise to the infant's central nervous system. Hyperinsulinemic hypoglycemia occurs in about 50% of infants who have BWS. In most, it resolves spontaneously. In a small group of patients, however, the hypoglycemia can be persistent and may require pancreatectomy.

The first line of treatment of hypoglycemia is the infusion of dextrose. The goal of therapy is maintenance of plasma glucose levels greater than 50 mg/dL at all times. Confirm low plasma glucose levels (<60 mg) obtained by portable glucometer with laboratory glucose analysis. At the time of hypoglycemia, obtain plasma ketones (acetoacetate and β-hydroxybutyrate), plasma fatty acids, serum insulin, and serum insulin growth factors (IGF-1 and IGF-2 by radioimmunoassay; large weight forms of IGF-2 can be detected by Western ligand blot).

Hydrocortisone analogous therapy is indicated when significant hypoglycemia is refractory to intravenous dextrose infusions.[23,24] If the infant cannot be weaned from dextrose, consider treating with diazoxide.[23] Evaluation by a pediatric endocrinologist is warranted for infants who have prolonged hypoglycemia lasting more than 1 week. Because the onset of hypoglycemia is occasionally delayed for several months, parents should be informed of the symptoms of hypoglycemia so that they can seek appropriate medical attention following discharge.

The infant's admission physical may reveal characteristic findings consistent with BWS, including ear grooves and pits, hemihyperplasia, and organomegaly. If structural abnormalities or tumors are suspected, MRI or CT examination of the abdomen is indicated. Treatment of neoplasias (tumor) can be accomplished in consultation with pediatric oncologist.

Accurate diagnosis of the infant who has multiple congenital anomalies is the most important step in patient care. The geneticists and genetic counselor are instrumental in putting the clinical features together to make the diagnosis of BWS. The correct diagnosis can lead to precise information for prediction of natural history (including reassurance), organization of appropriate laboratory studies, and the framework for health supervision and anticipatory guidance. The management plan can subsequently be used by the primary care provider following discharge.[20] Provide parents with resources and support group information (**Box 3**) and follow-up with the genetics clinic.

When the infant is well enough to begin oral feedings, evaluation by a feeding specialist may be needed to assist in overcoming feeding difficulties due to macroglossia. Specialized nipples, such as longer nipples used for infants who have cleft palate, or short-term nasogastric tube feedings may be needed to manage feeding difficulties. Infants who have enlarged tongues should be referred for follow-up with a craniofacial team, including plastic surgeons, orthodontists, and speech pathologists familiar with the natural history of BWS. Although tongue growth slows over

---

Box 3
National resources and support for Beckwith-Wiedemann syndrome

Beckwith-Wiedemann Support Network
   http://www.beckwith-wiedemann.org

Beckwith-Wiedemann Syndrome Children's Foundation
   Phone 425-338-4610
   http://www.beckwith-wiedemannsyndrome.org

Beckwith-Wiedemann Syndrome Family Forum
   http://www.beckwith-wiedemann.info/

BWS Registry
   bwsregistry@kids.wustl.edu

Family Village
   http://www.familyvillage.wisc.edu

time and jaw growth accelerates to accommodate the enlarged tongue, some children may benefit from tongue reduction surgery, typically performed between 2 and 4 years of age. Assessment of macroglossia related to speech difficulties by a speech pathologist may also be needed.

Infants who have structural renal abnormalities or gastrointestinal (GI) tract abnormalities need referral to the appropriate specialists. In some infants who have BWS, developmental anomalies of the renal tract are associated with increased calcium excretion and deposition (nephrocalcinosis). All individuals who have BWS should be screened for urinary calcium even when ultrasound findings are normal. A single random nonfasting urine sample obtained during hospitalization and at each health maintenance visit thereafter is recommended, and if abnormal a referral to a pediatric nephrologist should be given.

At the time of discharge referral for interventions, such as infant stimulation programs, occupational and physical therapy, and individualized educational programs, should be considered for infants who have BWS who may be at risk for developmental delay.

Consultation with an orthopedic surgeon is indicated if hemihyperplasia includes a significant difference in leg length. Surgery may be necessary during puberty to close the growth plate of the longer leg to equalize the final leg lengths. Referral to a craniofacial surgeon if facial hemihyperplasia is significant is also indicated.

Individuals who have BWS should be screened for Wilms tumor with ultrasound of the kidney every 3 months until 8 years of age.[25] Likewise, individuals who have BWS should be screened for hepatoblastoma with ultrasound of the liver. Ultrasound does not view the entire liver, however. Fortunately, serum AFP concentration is a marker for hepatoblastoma. At birth AFP levels are high and then gradually decline to adult levels by 10 to 12 months of age. A concerning AFP level is one that increases dramatically or one that does not decline during the first year of life. Dr. DeBaun[25] of the St. Louis Children's Hospital BWS registry recommends screening AFP measurements every 6 weeks up to 4 years of age. Unlike Wilms tumor the risk for hepatoblastoma drops off after age 4; therefore, ultrasound of the liver can be stopped after 4 years also.

The mode of inheritance in BWS is complex. Possible patterns include autosomal dominant inheritance with variable expression, contiguous gene duplication at 11p15, and genomic imprinting resulting from a defective or absent copy of the maternally derived gene. Both genetic (changing the structure of the gene) and epigenetic (influencing the function/expression of a gene without changing its structure) factors play a role.[2,24,26]

Genomic imprinting describes the process in which genetic material is expressed differently when inherited from the mother than when inherited from the father.[2,22,24,26] Human chromosome band 11p15.5 houses a large cluster of genes that are imprinted. Genes at chromosome band 11p15 are organized in two separately imprinted domains.

DMR1 contains several genes that encode proteins involved in growth regulation, such as paternally expressed IGF-2. DMR2 contains several imprinted genes, including the maternally expressed cell-cycle regulator cyclin-dependent kinase inhibitor (CDKN1C) and paternally expressed KCNQ1OT1 (L1T1) that regulates the expression of other genes in DMR2. Mutations in the CDKN1C gene can be found in 10% of the sporadic cases of BWS and 40% of the dominant cases. Loss of imprinted L1T1 accounts for 40% to 50% of cases of BWS.[2,24,26]

Currently, clinical testing is available for roughly 70% of the known mechanisms that produce BWS.[9] BWS occurs in monozygotic twins discordantly; the mechanism of discordance is unclear.[27-30] BWS occurs more frequently in pregnancies conceived with assistance of reproductive technologies.[31,32]

CASE REPORT TWO

A female infant who had prenatally diagnosed suspected meconium ileus was delivered by planned repeat caesarean section after labor began to a 25-year-old gravida 3 para 1 at 36 weeks and 5 days. Preconception and prenatal vitamins were taken. Maternal history included one prior healthy term pregnancy and a second pregnancy, 2 years previously, that had resulted in a ruptured bicornate uterus and yielded a stillborn at 22 gestational weeks. A prenatal ultrasound at 22 weeks' gestation identified a possible meconium ileus and calcifications and was significant for polyhydramnios. Group B streptococcus status was unknown at the time of delivery and the remaining prenatal laboratory studies were normal.

The infant presented with respiratory distress, grunting and retracting with decreased breath sounds bilaterally; physical examination was significant for a full and distended abdomen, which was tender on palpation with visible bowel loops, and bowel sounds were noted to be absent. Birth weight was 3.04 kg, length 47 cm, and head circumference 34.5 cm, all appropriate for gestational age.

Apgar scores of 6 at 1 minute and 8 at 5 minutes were assigned. The infant required continuous positive airway pressure by way of a mask intermittently over a period of 3 minutes and her oxygenation gradually improved. After initial stabilization, which included obtaining intravenous access, blood cultures, and a complete blood count and glucose level (which was 52 mg/dL) an Anderson tube was positioned in the stomach and placed to low intermittent suction before the infant was transported a short distance to the NICU, where surgeons had previously reviewed the prenatal ultrasounds.

On arrival at the NICU a chest radiograph was consistent with respiratory restriction secondary to impaired lung expansion related to peritonitis. An abdominal radiograph revealed multiple dilated loops of bowel seen in the upper and lower quadrants; scattered calcifications were seen in the left upper quadrant. The infant was intubated before going to the operating room after increasing respiratory distress and was extubated on day of life six. Subsequent physical examination revealed a grade 2 systolic ejection murmur and an ECG revealed a structurally and functionally normal heart, with an open patent ductus arteriosis. Routine admission screening showed serum glucose of 62 mg/dL after initiation of intravenous glucose administration at 80 mL/kg/d of a 10% glucose solution.

The infant was taken to the operating room on day of life 1, where a high jejunostomy and mucus fistula were created after 8 cm of bowel was resected. During surgery thick tenacious meconium and evidence of a congenital perforation were noted. A jejunostomy take-down and lysis of adhesions was performed on day of life 64. The infant did experience difficulty in reaching full-volume feeds post repair and was initially fed by way of jejunostomy tube and later transitioned to nasogastric and then to full oral feeds.

Sepsis evaluation initiated on admission was negative, although in view of surgery a full 7-day course of antibiotics (ampicillin and gentamicin) was completed. After the take-down surgery a 5-day course of ampicillin, gentamicin and metronidazole (Flagyl) was also completed.

In consultation with surgery and genetics, a work-up for CF was initiated. The infant was diagnosed with CF after two positive sweat chloride tests. Both parents of the infant tested positive for carrier status. The sibling of the infant was also tested and was found to be negative. The family received genetic counseling and after diagnosis the infant was referred to the CF and pulmonary clinics for further follow-up and ongoing management.

Discussion

CF is hereditary disease that affects the exocrine glands of the lungs, liver, pancreas, and intestines causing progressive disability and multiorgan system failure. The incidence of CF is 1:2500 in the white population and 1:17,000 in the African American population. CF affects whites five times more often than African Americans. CF is the most common, deadly, inherited disorder affecting whites in the United States. It is most common among individuals of Northern or Central European descent. CF is rarely seen in African Americans or Asians. Boys and girls are equally affected. Because there are more than 1000 mutations of the CF gene symptoms differ from person to person.

CF is an autosomal recessive disease, characterized by chronic obstructive lung disease, pancreatic exocrine deficiency, and elevated sweat chloride concentration.[33,34] Most children are diagnosed with CF by their second birthday. A small number of individuals are not diagnosed until age 18 or older, usually presenting with a milder form of the disease. Later presentation and diagnosis into adulthood is often related to infertility in males and females.

Absence of bowel movements in the first 24 to 48 hours of life may indicate CF. Between 10% and 20% of infants who have CF have meconium ileus, and 99% of infants who have meconium ileus have CF.[34,35] Meconium ileus is a failure to pass meconium, due to either mechanical obstruction or thickness of the meconium. The hyperviscous secretions from the mucous glands of the small intestine result in meconium that is thick and tenacious.[36] This process then can lead to an inability of the meconium to travel through the small intestine into the colon causing the ileum to become obstructed and at times perforate. An abdominal radiograph reveals dilated loops proximal to the obstruction; calcifications from previous perforations may be seen.[36] It is recommended to consider a work-up for CF in any infant who presents with meconium ileus.[20,27]

Signs and symptoms of CF in infancy and childhood include initial meconium plug, and distinctive stools—pale or clay-colored, foul smelling, or stools that float. In addition infants and children may have frequent diarrhea and fatigue, weight loss, or failure to thrive. They may have a salty taste to their skin. Infants and children may present with recurrent respiratory infection, such a pneumonia or sinusitis, and persistent coughing and wheezing.

CF transmembrane regulator (CTFR) functions as a cyclic AMP-activated chloride channel that allows for the transport of chloride out of the cell water molecules passively following chloride ions out of the cell, keeping secretions well hydrated. In CF an abnormality in CTFR blocks chloride transport. Inadequate hydration of the cell surface results, subsequently causing thick secretions and organ damage.

The gene that encodes for CFTR is found on the human chromosome 7, on the long arm at position q31.2. It contains about 170,000 base pairs. The encoded CFTR is a glycoprotein with 1480 amino acids. The protein consists of five domains. There are two transmembrane domains, each with six spans of alpha helices. These are each connected to a nucleotide-binding fold in the cytoplasm. These two nucleotide-binding folds are linked to a single regulatory R-domain that is a unique feature belonging only to this type of ABC protein.[34]

To date there is no cure for CF, although research is ongoing. Treatment is aimed at preventing complications, such as lung infections or digestive problems. How the condition is treated depends on the stage of the disease and the organs affected. Refer to **Table 5** for complications of CF.

An early diagnosis of CF and a comprehensive treatment plan can improve survival and quality of life. In a newborn, a screening blood test is used to test for the amount of a digestive enzyme (trypsin) in the blood. A high level shows the possible presence of CF. Many states now screen for CF on the Expanded Newborn Screening Test.

As the list of participating states is increasing it is recommended to check for participation with state health departments for inclusion.

When CF is suspected based on clinical presentation or diagnosis, evaluation follows a two-pronged approach. The first approach evaluates for a physiologic change of elevated chloride secondary to abnormal CTFR; however, this is not always possible in sick or premature infants. The sweat test is considered the gold standard for diagnosis. The second approach is aimed at identifying genetic mutations known to cause or to be associated with CF.

To perform the sweat test an infant must be greater than or equal to 36 weeks gestational age, weigh more than 2000 g and be at least 3 days of age. The sweat test is obtained after a collection device is placed on the infant's skin and a colorless, odorless chemical is applied to the skin (pilocarpine) that causes the infant to sweat. The test uses electrical-chemical stimulation of the skin to induce sweat (iontophoresis), which is then collected and analyzed for chloride levels. Elevated chloride levels are seen in infants who have CF. Two positive tests must be obtained to confirm diagnosis.

For those infants who do not meet the criteria because of their physiologic inability to produce sweat (ie, premature or small for gestational age infants), genetic testing is the second approach in confirming a diagnosis of CF. Because different laboratories have different protocols it is best to contact the facility that will be performing the testing for specific directions. ΔF508 is the most common genotype, occurring in up to 50% of patients who have classic CF. Most other CF mutations are rare; generally testing starts with the ΔF508 testing pathway and proceeds to the CF amplified for complete analysis of the CF gene. Positive results are returned in a 1-week time frame. Making an accurate early diagnosis is essential to optimizing management of this disease.

In the past, people who had CF were not expected to live beyond their teens. Today, CF is diagnosed earlier and treated more aggressively and effectively. As a result, people live fuller lives into their 30s, 40s, and beyond. An early diagnosis of CF and a comprehensive treatment plan can improve survival and quality of life. Specialty clinics for CF are helpful and can be found in many communities. Families who have a child diagnosed with CF and the children themselves need psychologic and social support because they may not be able to participate in normal childhood activities and may feel isolated.

The treatment of CF encompasses many body systems and includes antibiotics for respiratory

Table 5
Complications of cystic fibrosis by system

Respiratory	Recurrent bronchitis
	Recurrent pneumonia
	Pneumothorax
	Hemoptysis
Gastrointestinal	Pancreatic insufficiency
	Steatorrhea
	Decreased Vitamin A, E, D, and K levels
	Hepatobiliary disease
	Cirrhosis of the liver in advanced disease
	Esophageal varices
	Splenomegaly
	Hypersplenism
Reproductive	Infertility males due to congenital absence or atresia of vas deferens
	Infertility females due to thick tenacious mucous that occludes the cervical os
Endocrine	Diabetes mellitus

Box 4
Resources and support for cystic fibrosis

Cystic Fibrosis Support Group—Daily Strength

http://www.dailystrength.com/

Cystic Fibrosis.com

http://www.cysticfibrosis.com

International Cystic Fibrosis Support Group

http://cf.conncoll.edu

Reducing Isolation: an adult cystic fibrosis support group

http://www.videos.med.wisc.edu/videoInfo.php

Cystic Fibrosis Diagnosis and Support

http://www.mayoclinic.com

---

infections and bronchodilator therapy. Pancreatic enzymes are given to replace those not produced to aid with digestion. In addition, specific vitamin supplements, especially vitamins A, D, E, and K, are needed. DNAse enzyme replacement therapy is prescribed to thin mucus, making it easier to expectorate. Research has shown that the pain reliever ibuprofen may slow lung deterioration in some children who have CF. The results are most dramatic in children aged 5 to 13 years. Daily postural drainage and chest percussion to help mobilize secretions are also a standard of care. Heart and lung or lung transplant may be considered in some cases in end-stage disease. Infants and toddlers should have recommended immunizations as part of their regular care.

After diagnosis parents are provided with resources and support group information (**Box 4**) and follow-up with the genetics clinic. The primary care physician is a key member of the team and is often the gatekeeper for all care.[11,27] It is therefore essential that the primary care provider be identified and become involved in the infant's care as soon after diagnosis as possible. Families are offered ongoing genetic counseling and followed closely by CF clinics throughout their life span.

SUMMARY

Genetic conditions as a group are common and are a significant cause of mortality and morbidity.[4] In conditions involving a genetic component, as in all of medicine, accurate diagnosis is the most important step in patient care. The process of diagnosing a genetic disorder requires an evidence-

based approach applied to a sequence of events. After a specific diagnosis has been determined the next step, genetic counseling, can be initiated. Central to the team approach is always the concept of the family and the specific needs identified when a genetic disorder is diagnosed.

REFERENCES

1. Cassidy SB, Allanson JE. Management of genetic syndromes. Hoboken (NJ): Wiley-Liss; 2005.
2. Jones K. Smith's recognizable patterns of human malformation. 6th edition. Philadelphia: WB Saunders; 2005.
3. Cummmings M. Human heredity: principles and issues. 8th edition. Monterey: Brooks/Cole Publishing Company; 2008.
4. Jorde LB. Medical genetics. St. Louis (MO): Mosby 2006.
5. Gelehrter TD, Collins FS, Ginsburg D. Principles of medical genetics. Baltimore: Williams & Wilkins; 1998.
6. Miller SM. Individuals, families, and the new era of genetics: biopsychosocial perspectives. New York: W.W. Norton; 2006.
7. Hoyme HE, Seaver LH, Jones KL, et al. Isolated hemihyperplasia (hemihypertrophy): report of a prospective multicenter study of the incidence of neoplasia and review. Am J Med Genet 1998;79: 274–8.
8. Avery GB, Fletcher MA, MacDonald MG. Neonatology: pathophysiology and management of the newborn. Philadelphia: Lippincott, Williams & Wilkins; 1999.
9. Elliott M, Maher ER. Beckwith-Wiedemann syndrome. J Med Genet 1994;31:560–4.
10. Weng EY, Moeschler JB, Graham JM Jr. Longitudinal observations on 15 children with Wiedemann-Beckwith syndrome. Am J Med Genet 1995;56:366–73.
11. Pettenati MJ, Haines JL, Higgins RR, et al. Wiedemann-Beckwith syndrome: presentation of clinical and cytogenetic data on 22 new cases and review of the literature. Hum Genet 1986;74:143–54.
12. Barr CL, Best L, Weksberg R. Linkage study in families with posterior helical ear pits and Wiedemann-Beckwith syndrome. Am J Med Genet 2001;104:120–6.
13. Best LG. Familial posterior helical ear pits and Wiedemann-Beckwith syndrome. Am J Med Genet 1991;40:188–95.
14. Viljoen D, Pearn J, Beighton P. Manifestations and natural history of idiopathic hemihypertrophy: a review of eleven cases. Clin Genet 1984;26:81–6.
15. Engstrom W, Lindham S, Schofield P. Wiedemann-Beckwith syndrome. Eur J Pediatr 1988;147:450–7.
16. Goldman M, Shuman C, Weksberg R, et al. Hypercalciuria in Beckwith-Wiedemann syndrome. J Pediatr 2003;142:206–8.

17. Borer JG, Kaefer M, Barnewolt CE, et al. Renal findings on radiological followup of patients with Beckwith-Wiedemann syndrome. J Urol 1999;161:235–9.

18. Choyke PL, Siegel MJ, Oz O, et al. Nonmalignant renal disease in pediatric patients with Beckwith-Wiedemann syndrome. AJR Am J Roentgenol 1998;171:733–7.

19. DeBaun MR, Siegel MJ, Choyke PL. Nephromegaly in infancy and early childhood: a risk factor for Wilms tumor in Beckwith-Wiedemann syndrome. J Pediatr 1998;132:401–4.

20. Jorde LB, Carey JC, White RL. Medical genetics. St. Louis (MO): Mosby-Year Book; 1995.

21. Slavotinek A, Gaunt L, Donnai D. Paternally inherited duplications of 11p15.5 and Beckwith-Wiedemann syndrome. J Med Genet 1997;34:819–26.

22. Waziri M, Patil SR, Hanson JW, et al. Abnormality of chromosome 11 in patients with features of Beckwith-Wiedemann syndrome. J Pediatr 1983;102:873–6.

23. Young T, Mangum B. A manual of drugs used in neonatal care. 20th edition. Montvale (NJ): Thomas Healthcare USA; 2007.

24. Online Medelian Inheritance in Man. Beckwith-Wiedemann syndrome. Available at: http://www.ncbi.nlm.nih.gov/entrez/dispomim.cgi?id=130650. Accessed July 8, 2008.

25. DeBaun MR, Tucker MA. Risk of cancer during the first four years of life in children from The Beckwith-Wiedemann Syndrome Registry. J Pediatr 1998;132:398–400.

26. GeneReviews. Beckwith-Wiedemann syndrome. Available at: http://www.geneclinics.org/profiles/bws. Accessed July 8, 2008.

27. Marcus-Soekarman D, Hamers G, Velzeboer S, et al. Mosaic trisomy 11p in monozygotic twins with discordant clinical phenotypes. Am J Med Genet A 2004;124:288–91.

28. Olney AH, Buehler BA, Waziri M. Wiedemann-Beckwith syndrome in apparently discordant monozygotic twins. Am J Med Genet 1988;29:491–9.

29. Weksberg R, Shuman C, Caluseriu O, et al. Discordant KCNQ1OT1 imprinting in sets of monozygotic twins discordant for Beckwith-Wiedemann syndrome. Hum Mol Genet 2002;11:693–8.

30. Yoon G, Beischel LS, Johnson JP, et al. Dizygotic twin pregnancy conceived with assisted reproductive technology associated with chromosomal anomaly, imprinting disorder, and monochorionic placentation. J Pediatr 2005;146:565–7.

31. Chang AS, Moley KH, Wangler M, et al. Association between Beckwith-Wiedemann syndrome and assisted reproductive technology: a case series of 19 patients. Fertil Steril 2005;83:349–54.

32. DeBaun MR, Niemitz EL, Feinberg AP. Association of in vitro fertilization with Beckwith-Wiedemann syndrome and epigenetic alterations of LIT1 and H19. Am J Hum Genet 2003;72:156–60.

33. Schwartz MW. The 5-minute pediatric consult. Philadelphia: Wolters Kluwer Health/Lippincott Williams & Wilkins; 2008.

34. Tsui LC. Mutations and sequence variations detected in the cystic fibrosis transmembrane conductance regulator (CFTR) gene: a report from the Cystic Fibrosis Genetic Analysis Consortium. Hum Mutat 1992;1:197–203.

35. McGahren ED, Wilson WG. Pediatrics recall. Philadelphia: Lippincott Williams & Wilkins; 2008.

36. Longobucco DB, Ruth VA. Neonatal surgical procedures: a guide for care and management. Santa Rosa (CA): NICU Book Publishers; 2007.

Antimicrobial Use and Bacterial Resistance in Neonatal Patients

Christine Domonoske, PharmD*,
Karen Severson, PharmD

KEYWORDS

- Premature infant • Neonate • Antibiotic
- Bacterial resistance

Neonatal patients are particularly susceptible to infections. Because it is difficult to ascertain the presence of an infection, a high index of suspicion is necessary in this population. Once a decision is made to treat, the choice of antibiotic or antibiotics, the dosing of the regimen, and the length of therapy can all have major impacts on morbidity and mortality. As newer antibiotics become available, evidence and dosing information for this patient population are typically lacking. Because of the lack of neonatal data, the number of antibiotics given to the premature infant is limited compared with the adult population. This article compares the pharmacokinetic differences between premature infants and adults. It will provide the rationale for using certain antibiotics (ie, penicillins, aminoglycosides, vancomycin, and cephalosporins) in premature infants. The mechanisms of action, mechanisms of bacterial resistance, and side effects of these antibiotics are described. Antibiotics that should be avoided in this patient population are also discussed. Finally, neonatal nursing strategies to encourage the proper use of antimicrobial therapy, and mechanisms to decrease bacterial resistance, are described.

NEONATAL PHARMACOKINETIC DIFFERENCES

Specific dosing requirements in premature infants must be considered when using antibiotics. First, to optimize the probability of response to antibiotics, unpredictable pharmacokinetic influences should be minimized. Because one of the first signs of sepsis in premature infants may be feeding intolerance, oral antibiotics are used infrequently. Similarly, intramuscular (IM) injections cannot be given routinely because premature infants have a limited amount of muscle mass. Medications given by this route may cause local tissue or nerve damage. In addition, unacceptable and variable rates of absorption may occur with intramuscular injections because of the shunting of blood flow away from the extremities, especially in a hypotensive infant. Because of these factors, the intravenous (IV) route is the preferred route when treating infections in most neonatal patients.

Once an antibiotic is administered, the distribution of the antibiotic throughout the premature infant's body differs from the distribution in an adult's body. Premature infants have a much larger percentage of total body water than adults. Antibiotics distributed into total body water will be distributed over a much larger volume compared with the adult's body and therefore require increased weight-based doses to achieve adequate serum levels (ie, aminoglycosides). Changes in the total body water volume status during the first week of life may require more frequent dosing adjustments and careful serum monitoring. Conversely, the amount of total body fat is minimal in premature infants compared with adults. Much smaller weight-based doses of medications that penetrate into body fat are needed in the premature infant. However, this precaution usually does not apply to antibiotics but rather, to medications such as

Department of Pharmacy Services, Children's Memorial Hermann Hospital, Memorial Hermann Texas Medical Center, 6411 Fannin Street, Houston, TX 77030, USA
* Corresponding author.
E-mail address: Christine.Domonoske@memorialhermann.org (C. Domonoske).

Crit Care Nurs Clin N Am 21 (2009) 87–95
doi:10.1016/j.ccell.2008.09.002

ccnursing.theclinics.com

sedatives and narcotics. On the positive side, maturational changes in the permeability of the blood–brain barrier make the treatment of meningitis less complicated than in adult patients.[1]

The reduced hepatic and renal function in premature infants may prolong the half-life of some antimicrobials, thus requiring smaller or less frequent dosing. The liver and kidney functions improve with advancing chronologic age.[1] For this reason, the gestational age and the postnatal age of the patient must be considered when choosing the dosing regimen. A standard dose or dosing interval cannot be applied to all neonatal patients. Because most of the antibiotics given to neonatal patients are renally eliminated, additional dosing adjustments must be made if any further renal dysfunction occurs, to avoid adverse effects and increased toxicity.

BACTERIAL RESISTANCE

It is important to optimize the use of antimicrobial therapy to decrease or prevent microorganism resistance. The development of resistance can be enhanced by an inappropriate duration of treatment (too short or too long), insufficient concentrations of antibiotic at the infection site or sites, an overwhelming number of organisms, and overuse/misuse of antibiotics. Because premature infants receive multiple courses of antibiotics throughout their long hospital stay, the potential for developing infections with multidrug-resistant organisms is high. Likewise, the development and spread of resistant organisms is becoming more problematic in both the health care and community settings.

When microorganisms are exposed to an antibiotic, they are classified as susceptible, tolerant (intermediate), or resistant. Susceptible organisms are killed when exposed to a therapeutic concentration of antibiotic for the appropriate duration of time. Tolerant strains survive, but do not thrive, in the presence of the antibacterial agent. Tolerance can develop when an organism is treated for an inappropriate length of time or with subtherapeutic concentrations of antibiotics and can be passed on to the next generation of microorganisms. Bacterial resistance to an antibiotic allows a microbe to remain functional and to thrive, even in the presence of the antimicrobial agent, resulting in treatment failure.

It is becoming increasingly common for bacteria to express multiple resistance mechanisms, which may further complicate treatment regimens and increase morbidity, mortality, and cost.[2] Bacteria may acquire tolerance and resistance in various ways, including biochemical and genetic methods.

Spontaneous genetic mutations may evolve and incorporate genetic resistance codes from other bacteria. Thus, new resistant bacteria may pass the resistance from generation to generation. Resistance mechanisms evolve to allow microorganisms to overcome the effects of any antimicrobial agent that has the ability to harm the organisms. Bacteria become resistant to antimicrobials through a few primary methods (**Table 1**).

The first mechanism of resistance is inactivation of the drug. This resistance occurs when the bacteria produce enzymes (ie, β-lactamases, acetyltransferases, phosphotransferases, nucleotidyltransferases, esterases, and adenylases) that are capable of destroying the antibiotic. For example, β-lactamase enzymes inactivate β-lactam antibiotics by hydrolyzing the amide bond in the β-lactam ring and thus inactivating the antibiotic.[3]

The second method an organism may use to become resistant is by decreasing the ability of the antibiotic to reach the site of action. One of the ways organisms decrease access is by changing the inner and outer bacterial cell membrane characteristics to hinder the ability of antibacterial agents to enter the bacterial cell and exert their effects (ie, alteration in porin channels of *Pseudomonas aeruginosa* for β-lactam antibiotics).

Another method to decrease intracellular antibiotic concentration is through the use of an active efflux pump. Efflux pumps, present in many organisms (ie, *P. aeruginosa*, *Escherichia coli* [*E. coli*]), export the antibiotic out of the cell.

Lastly, the production of a biofilm covering helps protect the microorganisms from antibacterial agents. Biofilms are made up of complex networks of bacteria attached to a surface and connected by an extracellular matrix that protects the bacteria within the biofilm from antibiotics. Because the antibiotic cannot easily penetrate the biofilm, the likelihood of treatment failure increases. For example, *Staphylococci* produce biofilm as a protective mechanism.[4]

Altering the drug target and inhibiting the binding of the antibiotic to the organism's target site is another resistance mechanism. Drug target alteration can be accomplished by altering ribosomal target sites (ie, *Pseudomonas* to aminoglycosides), cell wall precursor targets (ie, methicillin-susceptible conversion to methicillin-resistant *Staphylococcus aureus* [MRSA]), or target enzymes (ie, sulfamethoxazole/trimethoprim [Bactrim, Septra]). Protection of the target site or overproduction of the target also can prevent the antibacterial agent from exerting the therapeutic antimicrobial effect.

Lastly, metabolic bypass is a method of resistance whereby organisms develop alternate

Table 1
Antimicrobial resistance mechanisms

Mechanism of Resistance	Organisms Using Mechanism	Antibiotics Affected
Drug inactivation		
Hydrolysis (β-lactamase)	Staphylococcus, Enterococcus, Escherichia coli, Citrobacter, Enterobacter, Morganella, Providencia, Serratia, Salmonella, Shigella, Pseudomonas, Proteus, Klebsiella, Neisseria, Bacillus, Haemophilus, Acinetobacter, Bacteroides, Burkholderia, Stenotrophomonas, Streptomyces, Fusobacteria, Clostridia	β-lactams
Modification (acetyltransferase/ phosphotransferase/ nucleotidyltransferase/ esterase/adenylase)	Staphylococcus, Enterococcus, Pseudomonas, Serratia, Escherichia coli	Aminoglycosides Macrolides
Decreased accessibility		
Membrane permeability (inner/ outer membrane)	Pseudomonas, Enterobacter, Neisseria, Serratia, Klebsiella, Bacteroides, Campylobacter, Escherichia coli, Salmonella, Staphylococcus	Aminoglycosides β-lactams Chloramphenicol Fluoroquinolones Tetracyclines Trimethoprim
Active efflux	Escherichia coli, Enterococcus, Bacteroides, Shigella, Pseudomonas, Staphylococcus, Streptococcus	β-lactams Fluoroquinolones Macrolides Tetracyclines
Biofilm	Staphylococci	β-lactams
Altered target (ribosomal target sites/cell wall precursor targets/ target enzymes/protection of target site/overproduction of target)	Haemophilus, Neisseria, Escherichia coli, Pseudomonas, Enterococcus, Mycoplasma, Campylobacter, Staphylococcus, Citrobacter	Aminoglycosides β-lactams Chloramphenicol Clindamycin Fluoroquinolones Macrolides Rifampin Sulfonamides Tetracyclines Trimethoprim Vancomycin
Metabolic bypass	Staphylococcus, Enterococcus, Neisseria	Sulfonamides Trimethoprim

Data from McManus MC. Mechanisms of bacterial resistance to antimicrobial agents. Am J Health Pharm 1997;54(12):1420–33; and Cloutier MJ. Antibiotics: mechanisms of action and the acquisition of resistance – when magic bullets lose their magic. Am J Pharm Educ 1995;59:167–72.

metabolic pathways, preventing the antibiotic from acting on the primary target (ie, *P. aeruginosa* and fluoroquinolones).[2,5]

To decrease resistance, it is important for the neonatal practitioner to have an understanding of the antibiotics prescribed in this patient population. The most commonly administered antibiotics in the neonatal population are the penicillins,

aminoglycosides, vancomycin (Vancocin), and cephalosporins.

PENICILLINS

Several penicillins, also known as β-lactam antibiotics and including ampicillin, aqueous penicillin G (Pfizerpen), oxacillin, and nafcillin, are given to neonatal patients. Penicillins exert their antimicrobial action by binding to the bacteria's penicillin-binding proteins, causing lysis of the bacterial cell wall. These antibiotics are considered bactericidal because they cause the death of susceptible bacteria.

The most common antibiotic given to neonatal patients is ampicillin. This antibiotic is usually started immediately after birth if sepsis is suspected. Ampicillin covers two of the three most common organisms responsible for early-onset sepsis in the neonate (ie, group B Streptococcus and Listeria monocytogenes). In fact, women colonized with group B Streptococcus will receive ampicillin or penicillin prophylactically before delivery. This practice has greatly reduced the incidence of early-onset group B Streptococcus infections in the neonate. However, it also has resulted in the increased incidence of E. coli sepsis, which has surpassed group B Streptococcus as the most common organism causing early-onset neonatal sepsis. The widespread use has also led to the increasing resistance of E. coli to ampicillin.[6] Increased E. coli resistance has necessitated the addition of a second antibiotic to be given in combination with ampicillin if an infection is suspected shortly after birth. If only group B Streptococcus is cultured from the neonatal patient, the antibiotics can be converted to aqueous penicillin G, which is a more narrow spectrum antibiotic. An additional use of penicillin G is for the treatment of congenital syphilis.

A common pathogen causing late-onset infections in premature infants is S. aureus. Approximately 60 years ago, S. aureus was easily eradicated by penicillin G. Today, this bacterium has altered its penicillin-binding protein site to decrease the affinity of the β-lactam antibiotics to the organism,[7] rendering them useless. As such, vancomycin has become the preferred antibiotic over oxacillin and nafcillin for late-onset neonatal infections. However, if a methicillin-susceptible S. aureus infection is identified through culture and susceptibility results, oxacillin or nafcillin become the antibiotics of choice because of their bactericidal effects and narrower spectrum of action.

Both gram-positive and gram-negative organisms can produce β-lactamase enzymes, which hydrolyze the β-lactam ring found in the structures of penicillins and cephalosporins. Hydrolysis of this ring will render the antibiotic ineffective. For example, this type of resistance can occur with E. coli resistance to ampicillin and S. aureus resistance to penicillin G and ampicillin.

The side effects of the penicillin antibiotics are minimal. All penicillin antibiotics, except nafcillin, are renally eliminated. Because premature infants have immature kidneys with reduced renal function, doses must be given less frequently compared with older children and adults. If given too frequently, the chance of inducing seizures from high penicillin levels will be greatly increased. Although allergies to the penicillin antibiotics are common in adults, this occurrence is rare to nonexistent in the neonatal population (even if the parents have this history) because they cannot mount these types of reactions in their premature state.

AMINOGLYCOSIDES

Aminoglycoside antibiotics, which include gentamicin (Garamycin), tobramycin (Nebcin), and amikacin (Amikin), are another group of antibiotics used as first-line agents in neonatal patients. Aminoglycosides inhibit protein synthesis by irreversibly binding to the 30S ribosomal subunits, thus disrupting the outer bacterial cell membrane, resulting in cell death. Gentamicin, combined with ampicillin, is used immediately after birth to treat suspected infections resulting from gram-negative organisms, such as E. coli. When late-onset infections occur, either gentamicin or tobramycin can be used to treat nosocomial gram-negative organisms such as Pseudomonas, Enterobacter, or Klebsiella. Aminoglycosides are used in conjunction with β-lactam antibiotics to facilitate synergistic killing of gram-negative organisms such as Pseudomonas.[8] Amikacin is usually reserved for infections caused by organisms that are resistant to gentamicin and tobramycin, and therefore, it is used much less frequently.

Although aminoglycosides cannot be used as monotherapy for the treatment of infections caused by gram-positive organisms, gentamicin has synergistic activity against gram-positive organisms when combined with antibiotics targeting bacterial cell walls. For example, the addition of small doses of gentamicin causes vancomycin or ampicillin to become bactericidal against Enterococcus.[9]

Organisms appear to use three main mechanisms to develop resistance to aminoglycosides. One mechanism of aminoglycoside resistance is the alteration in the ribosomal target, thus preventing the ribosomal binding of the aminoglycoside. Production of enzymes that inactivate aminoglycosides are a second mechanism of resistance. Enzymes such as adenylase, acetyltransferase, and phosphotransferase are common examples and can affect any of the aminoglycosides. The last mechanism of resistance, alteration of the cellular transport system, results in decreased transport of aminoglycosides into the cell and affects all of the aminoglycosides equally.[10–15]

The two major side effects of aminoglycosides are nephrotoxicity and ototoxicity. Nephrotoxicity occurs in approximately 10% to 25% of adult patients but occurs less frequently in neonatal patients.[16] Aminoglycoside-induced nephrotoxicity is usually reversible and has been correlated with elevated trough levels or prolonged durations of therapy. Ototoxicity occurs in approximately 2% to 15% of all patients and is usually irreversible or only partially reversible. Ototoxicity associated with aminoglycosides has been correlated with prolonged durations of therapy.[17]

To maximize efficacy, aminoglycosides should be monitored using peak concentrations. Trough levels should be obtained to minimize the side effects. In the neonatal patient, it is important to obtain aminoglycoside levels for patients being treated for prolonged durations. Treatment durations of 3 days or less do not require serum monitoring, unless the patient has significant renal impairment. When serum levels are required, levels should be drawn around the third dose. A trough level should be drawn immediately before the third dose, and a peak level should be drawn 30 minutes after the end of a 30-minute infusion. If the patient has significant renal impairment, a trough level should be obtained before the second dose. The goal peak level will vary with the type of infection being treated. Because the aminoglycosides concentrate in the urine, the lower end of the peak therapeutic range is desired when treating urinary tract infections. For the treatment of sepsis or pneumonia, the upper end of the peak therapeutic range is required. When gentamicin is used as a synergistic therapy, peak levels slightly below the therapeutic range are appropriate (ie, 3–4 mg/dL). Trough levels should always be maintained within the therapeutic range (**Table 2**).

In the adult population, one aminoglycoside dosing strategy uses high aminoglycoside doses with extended dosing intervals. The rationale for this is to increase the efficacy of the aminoglycosides by obtaining high peak levels while minimizing toxicity by allowing the serum level to fall over an extended time frame. This strategy has been shown to be as effective as giving multiple doses per day and may be less toxic. Nevertheless, this dosing strategy has not been well studied in premature infants because of neonates' larger volume of distribution and decreased renal elimination of aminoglycosides. More studies are needed before this dosing practice becomes standard in the neonatal patients.[18]

VANCOMYCIN

Vancomycin is a glycopeptide antibiotic that binds to cell wall peptides, inhibiting peptidoglycan synthesis resulting in cell wall disruption. This disruption occurs at a different site, compared with penicillins or cephalosporins. Vancomycin is bactericidal for most gram-positive organisms, but is bacteriostatic against *Enterococcus* unless combined with gentamicin.[19]

Vancomycin was first isolated from the organism *Streptomyces* and was used to treat penicillin-resistant *S. aureus* infections before less toxic alternatives (ie, methicillin and nafcillin) were discovered. However, after years of using methicillin, nafcillin, and oxacillin, *Staphylococci* altered its penicillin-binding protein site to become resistant to these antibiotics. Today, vancomycin is used to treat MRSA infections. Mothers and health care workers may be colonized with MRSA, which may result in the spread of this organism to premature infants. Some neonatal intensive care units do routine MRSA screening cultures to isolate infants who are MRSA positive to prevent the spread of this organism.

The most common use of vancomycin in the neonatal population is to treat coagulase-negative *Staphylococci*, the most common cause of late-onset infections in the neonatal population, which have a high rate of resistance to all penicillins. The remaining use for vancomycin in the neonatal population is to treat infections caused by

Table 2	
Therapeutic antibiotic serum levels	
Antibiotic	**Therapeutic Level**
Amikacin	Peak: 20–30 mg/dL Trough: <10 mg/dL
Gentamicin and tobramycin	Peak: 5–10 mg/dL Trough: <2 mg/dL
Vancomycin	Peak levels are not recommended Trough: 5–20 mg/dL

Enterococci. Fortunately, vancomycin-resistant *Enterococcus* is rare in the neonatal population and most *Enterococci* infections can be treated with ampicillin. Therefore, once the susceptibilities are known, therapy should be de-escalated from vancomycin to ampicillin. Even though vancomycin resistance is uncommon in premature infants, vancomycin usage should be limited whenever possible to slow the development of vancomycin resistance.

Resistance to vancomycin is caused by plasmid-mediated modification of peptidoglycan. Because of the transferability of this resistance mechanism, vancomycin resistance from vancomycin-resistant *Enterococcus* can be spread to *S. aureus.*[20] Gram-negative organisms have intrinsic resistance to vancomycin caused by a decreased permeability of the outer membrane. Cross-resistance does not occur with β-lactam antibiotics because their site of action is different.[21]

Neither therapeutic efficacy nor toxicity has been proved to correlate with vancomycin serum levels.[22] Nevertheless, most practitioners still monitor trough levels to ensure the level is within the desired range. Additionally, this antibiotic is renally eliminated and trough levels need to be monitored in premature infants because of their impaired renal function. The therapeutic range for vancomycin trough levels is between 5 and 20 mg/dL.[23] When treating infections involving tissues that are more difficult for vancomycin to penetrate, such as the lungs or brain, higher trough levels (ie, 15–20 mg/dL) are desired. Trough levels between 5 and 15 mg/dL are usually appropriate for other infections (see **Table 2**). Peak levels should not be monitored because they have not been shown to correlate with efficacy or toxicity. A vancomycin trough level should be drawn when the serum level achieves a steady-state concentration, usually immediately before the third dose. A trough level may be obtained before the second dose if significant renal impairment is present.

When vancomycin was first developed, ototoxicity and nephrotoxicity were adverse effects. Currently, with better purification of the drug formulation, these adverse effects are rare. However, nephrotoxicity may still occur in patients concurrently receiving other nephrotoxic agents, such as aminoglycosides or amphotericin B. One possible vancomycin infusion-related reaction is called red man or red neck syndrome. This syndrome is caused by a release of histamine and results in flushing in the upper body, neck, and face, and potentially, a sudden drop in blood pressure. This reaction is not a true allergy and can be avoided if the infusion time is extended. It is uncommon in preterm infants because of their inability to mount this type of histamine reaction.[24]

CEPHALOSPORINS

The cephalosporin antibiotics, also known as β-lactam antibiotics, work in a similar manner as the penicillins. They inhibit bacterial cell wall synthesis by binding to the organism's penicillin-binding proteins, resulting in a bactericidal action. Cephalosporin antibiotics are divided into four groups (generations), based on their bacterial coverage. With each generation increase, the antibiotic becomes more broad spectrum (**Table 3**).

First-generation cephalosporins have the most activity against gram-positive organisms. These antibiotics are mainly used for surgical prophylaxis for procedures where skin flora is of concern (ie, ligations of patent ductus arteriosus, tracheostomy placements). Because they are not as bactericidal against *S. aureus* as oxacillin or nafcillin, they have

Table 3
Cephalosporin antibiotics used in neonatal patients

	Cephalosporin	Coverage	Neonatal Indications
1st Generation	Cefazolin (Ancef)	Gram-positive	Surgical prophylaxis for skin flora organisms
2nd Generation	Cefoxitin (Mefoxin)	Gram-positive, gram-negative, anaerobes	Surgical prophylaxis for bowel surgery
3rd Generation	Cefotaxime (Claforan) or ceftazidime (Fortaz)	Gram-positive, gram-negative	Nosocomial gram-negative infections, meningitis
4th Generation	Cefepime (Maxipime)	Gram-positive, gram-negative	Nosocomial gram-negative infections, meningitis

limited use in treating gram-positive infections in the neonatal population. The second-generation cephalosporins have increasing activity against gram-negative organisms and anaerobes, along with continuing gram-positive coverage. These antibiotics are used primarily for surgical prophylaxis but offer a broader coverage than the first-generation cephalosporins. Because the anaerobes in the gastrointestinal tract are covered, the second-generation cephalosporins (especially cefoxitin [Mefoxin]) are used for prophylaxis during gastrointestinal surgery. The third- and fourth-generation cephalosporins are used most frequently in the neonatal population. These antibiotics have an extended spectrum of activity, which includes gram-positive and gram-negative coverage. Therapeutic cerebrospinal fluid levels necessary to treat meningitis can be readily achieved. Nosocomial gram-negative organisms (ie, *P. aeruginosa*, *Klebsiella pneumoniae*) are usually killed by the third- and fourth-generation cephalosporins.

Cephalosporins, in general, are not first-line agents for neonatal patients. These antibiotics are more broad spectrum than other available antibiotics and, as a result, resistance can develop quickly with widespread use. For instance, combining ampicillin with cefotaxime (Claforan) for the treatment of early-onset neonatal sepsis has been shown to induce the development of resistant organisms at a much faster rate compared with ampicillin with gentamicin.[25] Another, more recent, problem caused by the overuse of cephalosporins has been the development of extended-spectrum β-lactamases. This type of resistance has been identified with *E. coli* and *Klebsiella* species, resulting in the resistance to the extended-spectrum cephalosporins (ie, third- and fourth-generation cephalosporins). Infections with these organisms are often multidrug resistant and can lead to increased mortality rates.

In addition to developing resistance quicker, the combination of ampicillin and cefotaxime during the first 3 days of life results in an increased mortality rate compared with ampicillin and gentamicin.[26] Cefotaxime may be preferred over gentamicin because of the decreased incidence of renal toxicity and the improved penetration into the cerebrospinal fluid. Hence, the increased mortality rate could be related to some other underlying factors, rather than the cephalosporin itself.

The use of extended-spectrum cephalosporin antibiotics has been associated with the development of invasive candidiasis in extremely low birth weight infants.[27] As a result, most clinicians reserve the use of cephalosporins for surgical prophylaxis or for patients who have infections caused by multidrug resistant organisms, meningitis, or severe renal dysfunction.

In general, the side effects of cephalosporins are benign. Although extremely rare, seizures could develop if the cephalosporin dosing intervals are not extended because of immature or reduced kidney function. In addition, transient bone marrow suppression may occur, resulting in neutropenia or thrombocytopenia.

ANTIMICROBIAL AGENTS TO AVOID IN NEONATES

Some antibiotics cannot be used in the neonatal population because of a lack of clinical trials proving their efficacy or a lack of clinical trials determining the most appropriate neonatal dosing regimens. Additionally, several antibiotics should be avoided in the neonatal population because of documented toxicities. The antibiotics that should be avoided include ceftriaxone, sulfamethoxazole/trimethoprim, and tetracycline derivatives.

Ceftriaxone (Rocephin) is a third-generation cephalosporin. This antibiotic should be avoided in infants younger than 2 months of age who have hyperbilirubinemia. Because of its high albumin binding, ceftriaxone will displace bilirubin from albumin binding sites, resulting in an increased risk for kernicterus. In addition, ceftriaxone should not be used in patients receiving IV fluids containing calcium. The Food and Drug Administration (FDA) has issued a warning regarding this concomitant use based on case reports of neonatal fatalities due to the precipitation of calcium with ceftriaxone. Fatalities have generally been associated with simultaneous IV administration, but administration at different times and through different infusion lines have also proved fatal. Recommendations from the FDA are to avoid administration of ceftriaxone and IV calcium-containing products within 48 hours of each other.[28] The only indication for ceftriaxone in the neonatal patient is for infants born to women who have untreated gonococcal infection. These infants should receive a single dose of ceftriaxone.[29]

Another antibiotic that should be avoided in patients younger than 2 months old is sulfamethoxazole/trimethoprim. Similar to ceftriaxone, sulfa-containing antibiotics compete with bilirubin for the albumin binding sites, which can cause displacement of the bilirubin and lead to an increased risk for kernicterus.[30]

Lastly, tetracycline derivatives (ie, doxycycline [Vibramycin], minocycline [Minocin], tetracycline [Sumycin] and tigecycline [Tygacil]) should not be used in patients younger than 8 years of age. If used during the period of tooth development, tetracycline derivatives may cause permanent tooth discoloration and enamel hypoplasia. In addition, in patients younger than 4 years of age or those receiving high doses, skeletal development and bone growth may be retarded.[31,32]

NEONATAL NURSING RESPONSIBILITIES

Neonatal nurses are in the best position to help prevent infections. They are the first line of defense when it comes to touching and handling the neonatal patients. Nurses should be empowered to enforce proper hand hygiene. Everyone should use alcohol-based hand cleansers before and after touching the patient. Likewise, sterile techniques should be used when cultures are obtained and when medications are being prepared or injected through the IV, IM or subcutaneous route to prevent contamination.

The timing of antibiotics is also critical. Once sepsis is suspected, antibiotics should be started within the first hour of diagnosis.[33] The nurse can help facilitate this by sending the antibiotic orders immediately to the pharmacy and following up if they are not received within a timely manner. The nurse can also ensure that all future doses are given at the appropriate time intervals to prevent untimely gaps in therapy.

Probably the most important function of the neonatal nurse is to double-check the doses of the antibiotics. Because suboptimal doses can promote resistance and high doses can lead to toxicity, it is important to give the correct dosing regimen. Unlike adult patients, one regimen cannot be used for most patients. Because the gestational age of the neonatal patient is needed to determine the dose and the interval of the antibiotics, the nurse must check that the correct regimen is written. In addition, the nurse should double-check the prepared dose by comparing the volume in the syringe with the medication's labeled dose to ascertain that the correct amount was prepared. It is also important to check the written order with the label to make sure that it was dispensed appropriately. Errors can easily happen during the ordering and preparation process. A double-check system helps limit potential errors and promotes patient safety.

Nurses spend the most time observing the patients and are some of the best judges of a patient's clinical status. Often, the physicians rely on the nurse's ability to determine if the patient is "acting normal." Although the culture results are an important determinant of the length of therapy, they may not tell the whole story if the patient was exposed to antibiotics in utero. Any information about the clinical status of the patient should be communicated to the physician before the final decision is made to stop the antibiotic or antibiotics. Although antibiotics should be discontinued as soon as possible, stopping the antibiotics before an infection is treated adequately can be detrimental.

Lastly, the nurse is responsible for ensuring that all antibiotic levels are drawn appropriately. Timing is essential. Levels drawn too early will be falsely elevated. Levels drawn late will be falsely low. To achieve the best dosing regimen, all blood samples should be drawn at the appropriate time. The time the levels are drawn and the time the dose is given should be documented accurately so the levels can be interpreted correctly and the regimens can be adjusted accordingly. Premature infants have a small circulating blood volume. Antibiotic levels that must be repeated because they were drawn at inappropriate times will increase the need for blood transfusions. Any unnecessary levels should be avoided, especially in patients on antibiotics for a short duration (ie, less than 3 days).

SUMMARY

The neonatal population is at extremely high risk for developing infections. Because of the premature infant's prolonged length of stay, these patients may receive several courses of antibiotics while hospitalized. Although the number of antibiotics used in this population is limited, the dosing regimens must be carefully prescribed and adjusted to account for changing pharmacokinetic parameters. In addition, the development of antimicrobial resistance should always be a concern. The neonatal nurse can help ensure that antimicrobial regimens are given appropriately and help monitor these regimens for efficacy, toxicity, and adverse effects.

REFERENCES

1. Kearns GL, Abdel-Rahman SM, Alander SW, et al. Developmental pharmacology – drug disposition, action, and therapy in infants and children. N Engl J Med 2003;349:1157–67.
2. Tenover FC. Mechanisms of antimicrobial resistance in bacteria. Am J Med 2006;119(6 Suppl 1):S3–10.
3. Krishna BVS, Patil AB, Chandrasekhar MR. Extended spectrum β lactamase producing Klebsiella pneumoniae in neonatal intensive care unit. Indian J Pediatr 2007;74(7):627–30.
4. Klingenberg C, Aarag E, Ronnestad A, et al. Coagulase-negative staphylococcal sepsis in neonates: association between antibiotic resistance, biofilm formation, and the host inflammatory response. Pediatr Infect Dis J 2005;24(9):817–22.

5. McManus MC. Mechanisms of bacterial resistance to antimicrobial agents. Am J Health Syst Pharm 1997;54(12):1420–33.

6. Bizzarro MJ, Dembry LM, Batimore RS, et al. Changing patterns in neonatal Escherichia coli sepsis and ampicillin resistance in the era of intrapartum antibiotic prophylaxis. Pediatrics 2008;121(4):689–96.

7. Dever LA, Dermody TS. Mechanisms of bacterial resistance to antibiotics. Arch Intern Med 1991; 151:886–95.

8. Song W, Woo HJ, Kim JS, et al. In vitro activity of beta-lactams in combination with other antimicrobial agents against resistant strains of Pseudomonas aeruginosa. Int J Antimicrob Agents 2003;21(1):8–12.

9. Babalola CP, Patel KB, Nightingale CH, et al. Synergistic activity of vancomycin and teicoplanin alone and in combination with streptomycin against Enterococcus faecalis strains with various vancomycin susceptibilities. Int J Antimicrob Agents 2004; 23(4):343–8.

10. Ristuccia AM, Cunha BA. An overview of amikacin. Ther Drug Monit 1985;7(1):12–25.

11. Moellering RC Jr. Rationale for use of antimicrobial combinations. Am J Med 1983;75(2A):4–8.

12. Phillips I. Good antimicrobial prescribing. Aminoglycosides. Lancet 1982;2(8293):311–4.

13. Bailey RR. The aminoglycosides. Drugs 1981;22(4): 321–7.

14. Gregory D, Hirschmann JV. Prudent use of the aminoglycosides. Postgrad Med 1978;64(3):97–104.

15. Moellering RC Jr, Wennersten C, Kunz LJ, et al. Resistance to gentamicin, tobramycin and amikacin among clinical isolates of bacteria. Am J Med 1977; 62(6):873–81.

16. Haughey DB, Hilligoss DM, Grassi A, et al. Two-compartment gentamicin pharmacokinetics in premature neonates: a comparison to adults with decreased glomerular filtration rates. J Pediatr 1980;96(2):325–30.

17. Fee WE Jr. Aminoglycoside ototoxicity in the human. Laryngoscope 1980;90(10 Pt 2 Suppl 24):1–19.

18. Contopoulos-Ioannidis DG, Giotis ND, Baliatsa DV, et al. Extended-interval aminoglycoside administration for children: a meta-analysis. Pediatrics 2004; 114(1):e111–8.

19. Saribas S, Bagdatli Y. Vancomycin tolerance in enterococci. Chemotherapy 2004;50(5):250–4.

20. Courvalin P. Vancomycin resistance in gram-positive cocci. Clin Infect Dis 2006;42:S25–34.

21. Jones RN. Microbiological features of vancomycin in the 21st century: minimum inhibitory concentration creep, bactericidal/static activity, and applied breakpoints to predict clinical outcomes or detect resistant strains. Clin Infect Dis 2006; 42:S13–24.

22. Cantú TG, Yamanaka-Yuen NA, Lietman PS. Serum vancomycin concentrations: reappraisal of their clinical value. Clin Infect Dis 1994;18(4):533–43.

23. Rybak MJ. The pharmacokinetic and pharmacodynamic properties of vancomycin. Clin Infect Dis 2006;42:S35–9.

24. Levine DP. Vancomycin: a history. Clin Infect Dis 2006;42:S5–12.

25. Bryan CS, John JF, Pai MS, et al. Gentamicin vs cefotaxime for therapy of neonatal sepsis. Am J Dis Child 1985;139:1086–9.

26. Clark RH, Bloom BT, Spitzer AR, et al. Empiric use of ampicillin and cefotaxime, compared with ampicillin and gentamicin, for neonates at risk for sepsis is associated with an increased risk of neonatal death. Pediatrics 2006;117:67–74.

27. Cotton CM, McDonald S, Stoll B, et al. The association of third-generation cephalosporin use and invasive candidiasis in extremely low birth-weight infants. Pediatrics 2006;118:717–22.

28. Ceftriaxone. Available at: http://www.fda.gov/CDER/DRUG/InfoSheets/HCP/ceftriaxone.htm. Accessed June 6, 2008.

29. Committee on Infectious Diseases American Academy of Pediatrics, et al. Gonococcal infections. In: Pickering LK, Baker CJ, Long SS, et al, editors. Red book: 2006 report of the Committee on Infectious Diseases. 27th edition. Elk Grove Village(IL): American Academy of Pediatrics; 2006. p. 308–9.

30. Bactrim package insert. Dee Why NSW (Australia): Roche Products Pty Limited; 2006.

31. Demers P, Fraser D, Goldbloom RB, et al. Effects of tetracyclines on skeletal growth and dentition. A report by the Nutrition Committee of the Canadian Paediatric Society. Can Med Assoc J 1968;99(17): 849–54.

32. Livingston HM, Dellinger TM. Intrinsic staining of teeth secondary to tetracycline. Ann Pharmacother 1998;32(5):607.

33. Dellinger RP, Carlet JM, Masur H, et al. Surviving sepsis campaign guidelines for management of severe sepsis and septic shock. Crit Care Med 2004;32:858–73.

Hyperbilirubinemia

Robin L. Watson, RN, MN, CCRN

KEYWORDS

- Hyperbilirubinemia • Jaundice • Kernicterus
- Phototherapy • Exchange transfusion

Hyperbilirubinemia is the most common condition requiring evaluation and treatment in newborns.[1] The clinical manifestation of hyperbilirubinemia—jaundice—occurs in 60% of normal newborns and nearly all preterm infants.[2–5] As compared with conditions such as persistent pulmonary hypertension of the newborn and congenital heart disease, which require advanced pharmacologic and technologic treatment strategies, hyperbilirubinemia seems to be overshadowed and may lose the attention it deserves as a condition that has potentially devastating effects. So severe are its consequences that the American Academy of Pediatrics (AAP) issued two practice guidelines[5,6] on the management of hyperbilirubinemia and the Joint Commission issued two sentinel event alerts[7,8] on kernicterus. Nurses must be vigilant when caring for babies with "just jaundice" by monitoring bilirubin levels, identifying infants at risk for developing severe hyperbilirubinemia, and implementing prescribed treatment effectively when indicated.

BILIRUBIN SYNTHESIS, TRANSPORT, CONJUGATION, AND EXCRETION
Synthesis

Bilirubin is produced by the breakdown of heme-containing proteins (**Fig. 1**). In newborns, 75% of all bilirubin comes from the catabolism of erythrocyte hemoglobin.[9] The remaining 25% of bilirubin is produced from the breakdown of other proteins, such as myoglobin, cytochromes, catalase, and peroxidases. Bilirubin synthesis starts with the lysis of senescent red blood cells (RBCs) in the reticuloendothelial system. When RBCs are degraded, heme is released from hemoglobin. Heme oxygenase, an enzyme found in most cells of the body except anucleated RBCs, catalyzes the first step in the breakdown of heme, yielding equimolar parts of biliverdin, iron, and carbon monoxide (CO).[10,11] Iron is conserved for new heme synthesis, and most of the CO is excreted by the lungs. From this initial step arise two points that have clinical implications discussed in more detail later: (1) Heme oxygenase is the rate limiting step for bilirubin production; inhibiting heme oxygenase limits the amount of bilirubin produced. (2) CO production is linked to bilirubin synthesis and, if measured, can serve as a proxy for the extent of hemolysis.

Biliverdin, a water-soluble, nontoxic, blue-green pigment is then rapidly converted by a second enzyme, biliverdin reductase, to indirect (unconjugated) bilirubin (4Z-15Z-bilirubin-IXa). This bilirubin isomer is orange-yellow, fat soluble, and not readily excreted in the bile or urine. Each gram of hemoglobin yields 35 mg of bilirubin.[9]

Transport and Hepatic Uptake

When released from the reticuloendothelial system, bilirubin is insoluble in water and must be transformed to a form that the body can excrete. Unconjugated bilirubin binds reversibly with albumin for its journey to the liver, where it is conjugated. The bilirubin-albumin (B/A) complex is vulnerable to separation by factors including metabolic derangements, such as acidosis and hypoxia, hypothermia, infection, and fatty acids. Drugs that decrease B/A binding include salicylates, sulfonamides, sodium benzoate, and indomethacin. The contribution that any of these make to creating severe hyperbilirubinemia is not thoroughly understood. Circulating bilirubin that is not bound to albumin is called "free bilirubin," which is the bilirubin that can enter the brain and cause neuronal injury.

Neonatal/Pediatrics, Harbor-UCLA Medical Center, 1000 W Carson Street, Box 14 Torrance, CA 90509, USA
E-mail address: rowatson@dhs.lacounty.gov

Crit Care Nurs Clin N Am 21 (2009) 97–120
doi:10.1016/j.ccell.2008.11.001
0899-5885/08/$ – see front matter

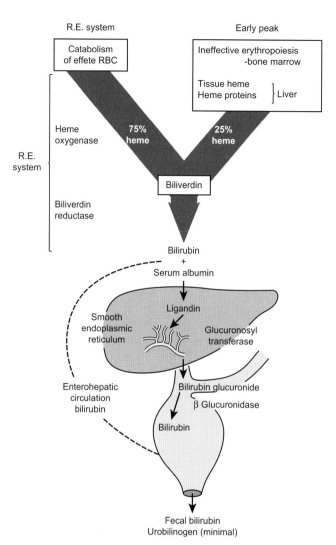

Fig. 1. Bilirubin synthesis, transport, and excretion. *Abbreviations:* RBC, erythrocytes; RE, reticuloendothelial. (*Adapted from* Maisels MJ. Jaundice. In: MacDonald MG, Mullett MD, Seshia MMK, editors. Avery's neonatology: pathophysiology & management of the newborn. 6th edition. Philadelphia: Lippincott Williams & Wilkins; 2005. p 770; with permission.)

Conjugation

When the B/A complex reaches the plasma membrane of the hepatocyte, bilirubin detaches from albumin and enters the liver cell. Inside the hepatocyte, bilirubin binds with other carrier proteins to be carried into the endoplasmic reticulum for conjugation. Protein Y is the primary carrier; protein Z is used during times of increased bilirubin load to the liver. Conjugation occurs inside the smooth endoplasmic reticulum, where each molecule of bilirubin combines with one or two molecules of glucuronic acid to produce bilirubin monoglucoronide and diglucoronide pigments. In children and adults, approximately two thirds of the monoglucuronides are conjugated to diglucoronides. In neonates, monoglucoronide is the predominate conjugate.[12,13] Conjugated bilirubin is water soluble and can be excreted into the bile and eventually eliminated from the body. Uridine diphosphoglucuronate glucuronosyltransferase (UGT) is the liver enzyme responsible for conjugation and formation of the glururonides. Sufficient supplies of glucose and oxygen are required for proper conjugation to occur.

Excretion

Once conjugated, bilirubin is readily excreted by the hepatocyte into the bile canaliculi as bilirubin mono- or diglucuronide. This water-soluble conjugated bilirubin is then emptied into the small intestine via the common bile duct. Conjugated bilirubin is not absorbed in the small intestine. The mono- and digluronides are relatively unstable molecules, however, and can be converted easily to unconjugated bilirubin and absorbed by the intestine. In the presence of mild alkaline conditions, such as exists in the jejunum and duodenum, and the nteric mucosal enzyme β-glucuronidase, conjugated bilirubin is hydrolyzed back to the lipid-soluble unconjugated form that is easily absorbed from the small intestine into the portal circulation. Enterohepatic circulation describes this route of circulation from the intestines to the liver and may explain why infants with gastrointestinal obstructions distal to the ampulla of Vater have hyperbilirubinemia.

Once conjugated bilirubin reaches the colon, it is catabolized by colonic flora to urobilinogen, some of which is oxidized to stercobilin, which is excreted in the stool. Stercobilin is what gives stool its brown color. Remaining urobilinogen is reabsorbed and excreted in the urine as urobilin. Urobilin is what gives urine its yellow color.

FETAL BILIRUBIN METABOLISM

Bilirubin can be detected in amniotic fluid after 12 weeks' gestation but disappears by 36 to 37 weeks' gestation.[9] The fetus has a limited ability to conjugate bilirubin. Circulating unconjugated fetal bilirubin readily crosses the placenta to the maternal circulation, where it is excreted by the maternal liver. Because fetal bilirubin is effectively excreted by the mother, newborns are rarely born jaundiced. Jaundice at birth usually indicates hemolysis, intestinal obstruction, or obstruction of the bile ducts.[9]

PHYSIOLOGIC CONSIDERATIONS IN THE NEWBORN

Unique aspects of normal newborn physiology transcend all steps of bilirubin metabolism and explain the jaundice seen in almost all newborns.

Increased Production

Newborns produce 8 to 10 mg/kg of bilirubin per day, more than twice the amount produced by adults.[14,15] The two primary reasons for increased production are a higher circulating RBC volume per kilogram and shorter RBC lifespan. Three fourths of bilirubin production comes from the breakdown of hemoglobin. Newborns have higher hemoglobin levels (17–19 g/dL)[16] and subsequently have a greater source for bilirubin production. The RBC lifespan in newborns is 80 to 100 days in term infants, 60 to 80 days in preterm infants, and 35 to 50 days in extremely low birth weight infants, versus 120 days in adults.[12] This decreased lifespan means faster breakdown of hemoglobin and an increase rate of bilirubin synthesis compared with adults.[11,12]

Decreased Transport and Hepatic Uptake

Albumin, bilirubin's ride to the liver, is like a bus. Newborns have fewer buses than older infants and adults. Plasma albumin levels are lower in newborns and inversely correlated with gestational age. Albumin levels increase by almost 30% over the first week of life but do not reach adult levels until 5 months of age.[17] Each "bus" also has a limited number of seats in which bilirubin can sit—binding capacity reflects the number of binding sites on the albumin molecule that can bind with bilirubin. Sick low birth weight babies have a diminished albumin-binding capacity (fewer binding sites) and are not able to bind as much bilirubin.[9] The extent to which decreased serum albumin and binding capacity affect neonatal hyperbilirubinemia is not thoroughly known. Once the seats on all the buses are full, any further increases in bilirubin (eg, hemolysis) leave bilirubin unbound and "free."

Inside the liver cell, bilirubin relies primarily on ligandin to be transported into the endoplasmic reticulum, where it is conjugated. Ligandin levels are diminished in the newborn and reach adult levels by approximately 5 days of life.[18] Fewer intracellular carrier proteins do not seem to be rate limiting, however.[9]

Decreased Conjugation

A major source of the normal hyperbilirubinemia seen in newborns is thought to be decreased activity of the UGT1A1 gene.[9] Glucuronyl transferase, the enzyme responsible for conjugation, depends on UGT1A1 activity. UGT1A1 activity is less than 1% that of adult values for the first 10 days after birth.[19,20] Adult levels are reached by 6 to 14 weeks of age.[20] Gestational age does not seem to influence the postnatal increase in UGT1A1 activity.

Decreased Excretion

Although not considered to be a significant rate-limiting step, the newborn liver has a decreased ability to excrete conjugated bilirubin and other anions, such as drugs and hormones.[9] During times of increased bilirubin load, the importance of this limitation heightens. Elevated serum conjugated bilirubin in the newborn may be seen for this reason when intrauterine hyperbilirubinemia occurs, as it does in isoimmunization.

Another mechanism that contributes significantly to newborn jaundice is an increased enterohepatic circulation, the result of increased β-glucuronidase activity, absent intestinal flora, and decreased intestinal motility. β-glucuronidase levels have been reported as being ten times higher in the newborn intestine than the adult intestine[21] and β-glucuronidase activity is higher in human milk than infant formulas,[22] which may contribute to breast milk jaundice. Intestinal flora are responsible for converting mono- and d-glucuronides to urobilinogen, which is either excreted in the stool or reabsorbed and excreted in the urine as urobilin. The lack of flora in the newborn intestine leaves conjugated bilirubin in the bowel and allows it to be deconjugated and available for recirculation. Although gut flora increase soon after birth, the flora found in the newborn intestine do not convert conjugated bilirubin to urobilin.[9,21] Intestinal motility is decreased in newborns, which increases the likelihood of bilirubin being unconjugated by beta glucuronidase. Infants who are fed earlier or fed more frequently have a lower incidence of jaundice. Infants who have meconium staining or who pass meconium early tend to have a lower incidence of jaundice.[23]

Physiologic Jaundice

Historically, the jaundice that occurs in most all newborns in the first few days of life has been termed "physiologic jaundice" and represents a phenomenon that occurs as a result of normal maturational limitations of the newborn. This term recently has come under scrutiny, however.[24] Maisels pointed out that many physiologic findings in newborns differ from those found in older children and adults. For example, newborns have faster heart and respiratory rates and lower blood pressure values. Just like bilirubin levels, these findings are related to maturation, yet the terms "physiologic tachycardia" and "physiologic tachypnea" are not applied.

The term "physiologic jaundice" also has been applied to newborns whose total serum bilirubin (TSB) falls within the normal range. Defining this normal range is problematic. The upper limit (95th percentile) of normal TSB has been shown to vary from 12.9 mg/dL to 17.5 mg/dL, depending on the population studied.[25–29] Because normal values of TSB vary in different populations, it is difficult to identify what is truly normal. Defining a finding as "physiologic" also implies that treatment is unnecessary. If left untreated, however, bilirubin levels within the "physiologic range" in premature infants are potentially hazardous and are treated with phototherapy. Maisels made a sound argument that in the neonatal intensive care population, the term "physiologic jaundice" has no meaning and no utility and should be abandoned.[9]

NATURAL HISTORY OF BILIRUBINEMIA

TSB levels in cord blood range from 1.4 to 1.9 mg/dL.[9] At birth, cord TSB levels are relatively normal because fetal bilirubin is cleared by the mother. After birth, the newborn has to assume responsibility for the process of conjugation and excretion. Because of maturational limitations in bilirubin conjugation and excretion, all newborns experience a rise and then a fall of TSB levels after birth. The rates of increase and decline in TSB and peak TSB level are affected by many factors, including gestational age, race, and breastfeeding. The advent of exchange transfusion and phototherapy adds to the difficulty of getting a true picture of the natural history of neonatal bilirubinemia because many infants with rising TSB levels are treated within 72 to 96 hours.

Bilirubin levels in normal term infants increase from birth, reaching peak levels of 5 to 7 mg/dL around days 3 to 5 of life and then decline by days 7 to 10.[21,30,31] Asian, Native American, and other populations of primarily breastfed infants have a much different pattern, with their peak levels being higher, reached later, and lasting longer.[9,21] Breastfeeding newborns have been shown to have mean peak TSB levels of 8 to 9 mg/dL.[29,32,33] Historically, a bilirubin concentration of 12.9 mg/dL was used as the upper limit of the normal bilirubinemia seen in newborns. This level was based primarily on data collected from the Collaborative Perinatal Project from 1955 to 1961, which found that 95% of infants had a TSB level lower than 12.9 mg/dL.[25] It is important to note that these data come from a time when 30% or less of mothers breastfed their infants. More recent data suggest that the upper limit of normal in the modern population is higher. In a review of 2840 infants, Bhutani and colleagues[27] found that the 95th percentile was a level of 17.5 mg/dL. Newman and colleagues[28] also found a TSB level of 17.5 mg/dL to be the 95th percentile in a review of 51,387 infants. Maisels and colleagues[9] reported the 95th percentile to be 15.5 mg/dL and 2 SD above the mean for TSB level to be 17 mg/dL in a study of infants in the United States, Hong Kong, Japan, and Israel. Maisels suggested that because of the consistency of these data, the modern upper limit of "normal" is a TSB level of 17 to 18 mg/dL.

Using contemporary data, Maisels and Kring[34] developed a nomogram indicating the velocity of increase in transcutaneous bilirubin (TcB) levels in a population of primarily breastfed North American newborns aged 35 or more weeks' gestation (**Fig. 2**). Smoothed curves for the 5th, 25th, 50th, and 95th percentiles are represented. Their nomogram does not replace Bhutani's hour-specific specific nomogram,[27] which is based on TSB values and is used to predict the risk of clinically significant hyperbilirubinemia. The nomogram

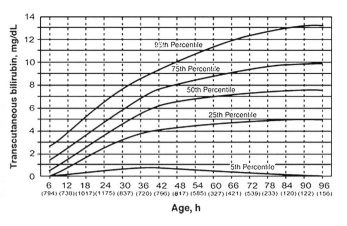

Fig. 2. Nomogram shows smoothed curves for the fifth, twenty-fifth, fiftieth, seventy-fifth, and 95th percentiles for TcB measurements among healthy newborns (gestational age: $\geq$ 35 weeks). A total of 9397 TcB measurements were obtained for 3984 newborns. The number of infants studied at each interval is shown in parenthesis. (From Maisels MJ, Kring E. Transcutaneous bilirubin levels in the first 96 hours in a normal newborn population of $\geq$35 weeks' gestation. Pediatrics 2006;117: 1170; with permission.)

may be useful for recognizing unusual trends and identifying infants who need additional evaluation or follow-up.[34]

BREASTFEEDING AND JAUNDICE

It is well established that breastfed infants have higher bilirubin levels than bottle-fed infants.[35–37] Breastfed infants are three times as likely to develop TSB levels higher than 12 mg/dL and six times as likely to develop TSB levels higher than 15 mg/dL as bottle-fed infants.[38] Although two phenomena associating breast milk and jaundice have been described—breastfeeding jaundice and breast milk jaundice—there is considerable overlap between the two entities and they may be indistinguishable from one another in some infants.[9] Breastfeeding jaundice usually begins within 2 to 4 days of life and peaks between days 3 and 6 of life. Approximately 10% of breastfed infants develop breastfeeding jaundice.[39] Various factors related primarily to the process of breastfeeding rather than the ingredients of breast milk may contribute to the development of breastfeeding jaundice. Dehydration, poor caloric intake, and increased enterohepatic circulation have been implicated in the cause of breastfeeding jaundice,[37] but increased enterohepatic circulation seems to be the primary mechanism responsible for this early-onset breastfeeding-associated jaundice.[22]

Breastfed infants take in fewer calories than bottle-fed infants, and an association between decreased caloric intake and an increase in the amount of bilirubin reabsorbed from the intestine has been shown.[40,41] Breastfed infants also pass less stool by weight and excrete significantly less bilirubin in their stools than do bottle-fed infants in the first 3 days of life.[42] Breastfeeding jaundice is managed not by limiting breastfeeding but by encouraging breastfeeding. Yamauchi and Yamanouchi[43] found that infants who nursed more than

seven times a day had lower bilirubin levels than infants fed fewer times a day. De Carvalho and associates[44] found similar findings with infants who nursed more than eight times a day compared with infants who nursed fewer than eight times a day. Improving milk intake by increasing feedings results in increased caloric intake, increased weight gain, increased meconium passage, and lower bilirubin levels and is strongly encouraged by the AAP.[6,43,44]

The second form of jaundice reported in otherwise healthy breastfed infants is breast milk jaundice. Occurring later, breast milk jaundice usually appears around days 4 to 7 of life and peaks between days 5 and 15 of life. Several theories exist to explain this pattern of jaundice, yet none has been confirmed unequivocally. It is believed, however, that the ingredients found in breast milk are the primary basis for breast milk jaundice. Early hypotheses proposed that substances found in breast milk, particularly pregnane-3α,20β-diol (a steroid metabolite of progesterone) and free fatty acids, inhibit UGT activity and interfere with bilirubin conjugation. There has been little evidence to support this theory, however.[22] The most likely mechanism is thought to be related to increased intestinal absorption of bilirubin into the enterohepatic circulation.[22] β-glucuronidase activity is higher in breast milk than formula and may play a role in breast milk jaundice. Bile salt-stimulated lipase, found in human milk, increases fat absorption, which is believed to be associated with an increased absorption of intestinal bilirubin. Decreased formation of urobilinogen found in breastfed infants also may play a role in breast milk jaundice. Infants fed breast milk excrete urobilin in their stools later than formula-fed infants.[9] Intestinal flora found in infants who are fed breast milk differs from those fed formula.[45] This difference may be responsible for the slower formation of urobilin and increased resorption of bilirubin in the intestine.[9]

UNCONJUGATED HYPERBILIRUBINEMIA

Serum bilirubin concentration is determined by bilirubin production or bilirubin load on the liver and bilirubin clearance excretion from the body. Any infant who is jaundiced in the first 24 hours should have a bilirubin level evaluated by either TSB or TcB.[6] When TSB concentrations reach levels higher than hour-specific normal values (**Fig. 3**), pathologic causes should be investigated. The following list identifies the causes of indirect hyperbilirubinemia in newborns:[9]

> Increased production or bilirubin load on the liver
>> Hemolytic disease
>>> Immune mediated
>>> Rh isoimmunization, ABO or other blood group incompatibilities
>> Heritability
>> Red cell membrane defects
>> Hereditary spherocytosis, elliptocytosis, pyropoikilocytosis, stomatocytosis
>> Red cell enzyme defects
>>> Glucose-6-phosphate dehydrogenase deficiency, pyruvate kinase deficiency, other erythrocyte enzyme deficiencies
>> Hemoglobinopathies
>>> α-Thalassemia, β-thalassemia
>> Unstable hemoglobin levels
>>> Congenital Heinz body hemolytic anemia
>> Other causes of increased production
>>> Sepsis
>>> Disseminated intravascular coagulation (DIC)

> Extravasation of blood, hematomas, and pulmonary, abdominal, cerebral, or other occult hemorrhage
> Polycythemia
> Macrosomic infants of mothers who have diabetes
> Increased enterohepatic circulation
>> Breast milk jaundice
>> Pyloric stenosis
>> Small or large bowel obstruction or ileus
> Decreased clearance
>> Prematurity
>> Glucose-6-phosphate dehydrogenase deficiency, pyruvate kinase deficiency
> Inborn errors of metabolism
>> Crigler-Najjar syndrome, types I and II
>> Gilbert syndrome
>> Galactosemia
>> Tyrosinemia
>> Hypermethionemia
>> Metabolic
>> Hypothyroidism
>> Hypopituitarism

Increased Bilirubin Production or Load on the Liver

The most frequently identified pathologic cause leading to hyperbilirubinemia is hemolytic disease of the newborn.[16] Fetal and newborn RBC destruction most commonly results from Rh or ABO incompatibility. Rh isoimmunization requires an Rh-negative woman who has developed antibodies to the Rh antigen and an Rh-negative fetus.

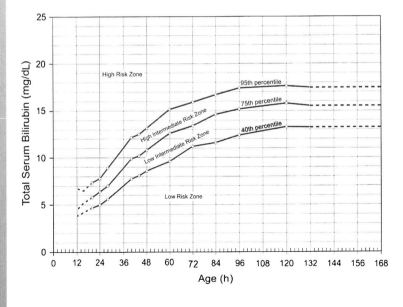

Fig. 3. Risk designation of term and near-term well newborns based on their hour-specific serum bilirubin values. The risk zone is designated by the 95th percentile track. The intermediate-risk zone is subdivided into upper- and lower-risk zones by the 75th percentile track. The low-risk zone has been electively and statistically defined by the 40th percentile tract. (Dotted extensions are based on < 300 TSB values/epoch). (*From* Bhutani VK, Johnson L, Sivieri EM. Predictive ability of a predischarge hour-specific serum bilirubin for subsequent significant hyperbilirubinemia in healthy term and near-term newborns. Pediatrics 1999;103:9; with permission.)

Development of antibodies to the Rh antigen takes place after exposure to Rh-positive blood, which can occur from an improperly matched blood transfusion or fetal-maternal blood transfusion during pregnancy, abortion, amniocentesis, or delivery. The IgG antibodies cross the placenta and destroy fetal Rh-positive RBCs. The antenatal administration of anti-D immunoglobulin (eg, Rho-GAM) to Rh-negative women has significantly decreased the incidence of Rh disease. Unlike Rh disease, ABO incompatibility does not require previous exposure to a different blood type. ABO incompatibility is seen in mothers who are type O and infants who are type A or B. Individuals with group O blood have naturally occurring IgG antibodies to group A and B, which can cross the placenta and destroy fetal RBCs. Naturally occurring antibodies found in mothers with type A or type B blood are mostly IgM antibodies, which do not cross the placenta. ABO blood group incompatibility is the most frequent cause of hemolytic disease in newborns; however, the disease is generally milder than Rh disease.[46] Minor blood group incompatibilities account for a small portion of infants with hemolytic disease.

Of the inherited diseases causing hemolytic disease in newborns, glucose-6-phophate dehydrogenase (G6PD) deficiency has received considerable attention recently as an important cause of neonatal hyperbilirubinemia.[7,47,48] G6PD is an enzyme found in all cells of the body, and it plays a significant role in protecting cells, especially RBCs, from oxidative damage. In the absence of G6PD, cells become vulnerable to oxidation resulting in cellular death. Hemolysis and hyperbilirubinemia in G6PD deficiency can be triggered by oxidative stress brought on by sepsis and exposure to several agents, including naphthalene (found in moth balls), agents used for umbilical cord antisepsis, breast milk of mothers who have eaten fava beans, and household cleaning agents.

G6PD deficiency is an X-linked disorder and the most common enzyme deficiency known; it affects 200 to 400 million people worldwide.[49] Population groups most affected include African, Southern European, Middle Eastern, including Mediterranean, and Asian. Although the overall incidence of G6PD deficiency in the United States is low (0.5%–2.9%),[50] it has been recently implicated as an important cause of kernicterus. Johnson and associates[51] reported that of 80 infants with kernicterus, 19 (24%) had G6PD deficiency. Twelve (63.2%) of these infants were African American. Although traditionally not much attention has been paid to G6PD in North America, G6PD deficiency is currently recognized as an important cause of neonatal hyperbilirubinemia and kernicterus.

Decreased Bilirubin Clearance

Conjugation of bilirubin inside the hepatocyte depends on a single form of the uridine diphosphoglucuronate glucoruonosyltransferase (UGT) enzyme. Three inherited defects of UGT deficiency are noted to cause neonatal hyperbilirubinemia: Crigler-Najjar syndrome types I and II and Gilbert syndrome.

Crigler-Najjar syndromes I and II are caused by one or more mutations of the five exons of the *UGT1A1* gene, the gene that determines the structure of UGT, or mutations in the noncoding region of the gene. Infants with Crigler-Najjar syndrome type I have no functioning UGT and are unable to conjugate bilirubin. Severe, prolonged unconjugated hyperbilirubinemia begins in the first few days of life and persists throughout life. Bilirubin levels are usually 20 to 45 mg/dL or higher.[52] These infants often require exchange transfusion in the first week of life.[9] Currently, the only definitive therapy for type I is liver transplantation. Human hepatocyte transplantation (infusion of liver cells into the portal vein) and administration of tin-protoporphyrin, tin-mesoporphyrin, and calcium phosphate have been used with limited success to reduce TSB levels.[53–57] Infants with Crigler-Najjar syndrome type II are able to synthesize small amounts of UGT and usually have less severe hyperbilirubinemia. Peak levels are 6 to 20 mg/dL, but they may be higher in newborns, and kernicterus has been reported.[9,52] Infants with type II generally respond well to phenobarbital therapy.

Gilbert syndrome occurs in approximately 6% to 9% of the population and involves a mutation in the *UGT1A1* gene promoter[9] or missense mutations in the coding region. Both autosomal dominant and recessive patterns of inheritance have been noted.[9] Individuals with Gilbert syndrome have reduced activity of UGT. Gilbert syndrome is most commonly diagnosed in young adults; however, neonates who are homozygous for the variant 7/7 UGT gene promoter have been shown to have a more rapid rise in TSB levels and higher TSBs than neonates without this variant.[58,59] When Gilbert syndrome occurs in combination with other conditions that exacerbate bilirubinemia, such as breastfeeding, G6PD deficiency, and blood group incompatibility, the risk of hyperbilirubinemia dramatically increases.[9]

CONJUGATED HYPERBILIRUBINEMIA

Elevated serum levels of conjugated bilirubin are a less frequent but significant cause of hyperbilirubinemia in neonates. Conjugated hyperbilirubinemia is the primary manifestation of neonatal cholestasis and should be differentiated from unconjugated hyperbilirubinemia.[6,60,61] Any infant who is jaundiced beyond 3 weeks of life should have a measurement of total and direct bilirubin levels and be evaluated for neonatal chole-stasis.[6,60,62] Neonatal cholestasis is defined as decreased canalicular bile flow and is a term used to describe various disorders associated with conjugated hyperbilirubinemia.[31,60] Subse-quently, biliary substances, such as bilirubin, bile acids, and cholesterol accumulate in the blood and extrahepatic tissues.

Neonatal cholestasis occurs in approximately 1 in 2500 live births.[60,62] Causes of neonatal cholestasis are extensive and described elsewhere.[61,62] Etio-logic factors can be classified based on the anatomic location of the pathology into extrahepatic or intrahepatic causes. Common extrahepatic causes are biliary atresia and choledochal cyst. In-trahepatic causes include idiopathic neonatal hepatitis, infections, α1-antitrypsin deficiency, and metabolic disorders, such as galactosemia, tyrosi-nemia, and glycogen storage disease type IV. Biliary atresia and idiopathic neonatal hepatitis are the most common causes of neonatal cholestasis.[60,61]

Because several disorders that cause neonatal cholestasis require immediate intervention for optimal survival, early recognition of cholestasis and prompt intervention are imperative. McKiernan[62] suggested a systematic and struc-tured approach to determining the cause, begin-ning first with evaluating the infant for conditions that require immediate intervention, such as sepsis, and metabolic disturbances, such as galactosemia and glycogen storage disorders. Once these causes have been ruled out, the next step is to investigate for biliary atresia. If a diag-nosis of biliary atresia is made, a Kasai portoenter-ostomy must be performed before the infant is 60 days old. If biliary atresia is ruled out, then the further evaluation to identify the cause ensues. Idiopathic neonatal hepatitis occurs in approxi-mately 15% to 30% of cases and is diagnosed when no specific cause can be found. As research continues to make progress in the areas of genetic and molecular basis of bile acid synthesis and transport, however, fewer infants are being placed into this diagnostic category. For more detailed information on unconjugated hyperbilirubinemia, the reader is encouraged to examine recent reviews of this subject.[60–62]

KERNICTERUS
Bilirubin Toxicity

The term "kernicterus" was first used more than a century ago to describe the yellow staining of the brain in the "kern" or nuclear region.[63]

Although originally used to describe pathologic findings of bilirubin staining of the brain stem nuclei, kernicterus has been used to describe acute and chronic effects of hyperbilirubinemia. To further confound important distinctions of the effects of bilirubin toxicity, the terms "kernicterus" and "bilirubin encephalopathy" have been used interchangeably. In an effort to bring greater clarity and consistency to definitions, the AAP[6] suggests that the term "acute bilirubin encephalopathy" be used to describe the acute manifestations of bili-rubin toxicity seen in the first few weeks of life and that the term "kernicterus" be reserved for describing the chronic and permanent clinical sequelae of bilirubin toxicity.

Recently, the term "bilirubin-induced neurologic dysfunction" has been coined to describe the changes associated with acute bilirubin encepha-lopathy along with a scoring system to quantify the severity of the symptoms.[64] Summarizing case reports that spanned more than 30 years, the AAP Subcommittee on Hyperbilirubinemia[65] concluded that kernicterus has a mortality rate of at least 10% and long-term morbidity rate of at least 70%. Kernicterus is recognized as a prevent-able life-long neurologic syndrome caused by severe and untreated hyperbilirubinemia during the neonatal period.[47]

Pathophysiology

Areas of the brain most commonly affected by bilirubin staining are the basal ganglia, particularly the globus pallidus and subthalmic nucleus, hippocampus, substantia nigra, cranial nerve nuclei, especially the occulomotor, vestibular, cochlear, and facial nerve nuclei, other brain stem nuclei, and the anterior horn cells of the spinal cord. These areas of neuronal injury help explain the clinical manifestations of bilirubin encephalopathy.

Just how bilirubin enters the brain is still not thor-oughly understood. Various theories exist to support bilirubin transport across an intact blood-brain barrier and across a damaged blood-brain barrier. The sulfisoxazole tragedy of the late 1950s gave rise to the hypothesis that free bilirubin, that portion of bilirubin not bound to albumin, crosses the intact blood-brain barrier and causes neuronal injury.[66] Odell[67] showed that sulfisoxazole and bilirubin compete for plasma albumin binding sites, thereby increasing the amount of free bilirubin. Benzyl alcohol, a preservative added to solutions of normal saline in the 1970s, may have caused kernicterus by the same mechanism.[68] Entry across an intact blood-brain barrier likely occurs by bilirubin binding with phospholipids of capillary endothelial cells, which then easily move into the brain. Anything that overwhelms the ability of bilirubin to bind with albumin, such as increased synthesis of bilirubin, decreased albumin levels, or competition for binding sites, can lead to increased amounts of free bilirubin and would be expected to enhance the movement of bilirubin into the brain. These bilirubin-phospholipid complexes are also relatively unstable.

Bilirubin tends to take up hydrogen ions, forming aggregates of toxic bilirubin acid that may damage the capillary endothelial cell and may advance the further uptake of bilirubin by the brain.[69] This occurrence may explain why acidosis may play a role in bilirubin encephalopathy because bilirubin acid is enhanced in an acidotic environment. Evidence also exists to suggest that bilirubin, still bound to albumin, crosses a damaged blood-brain barrier.[69] Bilirubin still needs to dissociate from albumin, however, to cause neuronal toxicity. Hyperosmolar solutions, hypercarbia, asphyxia, intracranial infection, and increases in blood pressure are known to pose risks to the blood-brain barrier and may play a role in bilirubin encephalopathy.[69] The mechanism of injury to neurons is also not thoroughly understood; however, it is likely that injury to cellular membranes plays a significant role.[69] Volpe proposed that free bilirubin enters intracellular organelles, such as mitochondria, endoplasmic reticulum, and nucleus, in a similar way that free bilirubin gained access to the brain by binding to membrane phospholids. In the brain, the susceptibility to injury varies by cell type, brain maturity, and brain metabolism.

Traditionally, a peak serum bilirubin level of more than 20 mg/dL has been used to predict a poor outcome in infants with Rh hemolytic disease.[70] In otherwise healthy neonates without hemolytic disease, serum bilirubin levels that do not exceed 25 mg/dL are unlikely to place these infants at risk of adverse neurodevelopmental consequences.[9,71] It is not possible to establish a TSB level that is safe for all infants, however, because of the multitude of factors that may influence bilirubin's ability to enter the brain.

Signs and Symptoms

Acute encephalopathy usually progresses through three phases, each of increasing severity.[69] The first phase occurs in the first few days and is characterized by slight stupor (lethargy, sleepiness, slight hypotonia, decreased movement, and poor sucking). Infants who are not managed effectively at this phase show a significant deterioration in prognosis.[69] After a week, the cardinal signs of the second phase appear, including marked stupor, often with irritability, increased tone, fever, and

a high-pitched cry. The increased tone is demonstrated by backward arching of the neck (retrocollis) and trunk (opisthotonus), rigid extension of all four extremities, tight-fisted posturing of the arms, and crossed extension of the legs. Subsequently, phase three is characterized by deep stupor or coma, increased tone, pronounced retrocollis and opisthotonus, no feeding, and a shrill cry.

Chronic bilirubin encephalopathy, kernicterus, is demonstrated by a tetrad consisting of extrapyramidal disturbances, auditory abnormalities, gaze palsies, and dental dysplasia.[9] These manifestations may not become apparent until after 6 months to 1 year of age.[69] Extrapyramidal movement abnormalities are the most remarkable feature of the tetrad and may not be well developed for several years. The most prominent motor movement is athetosis, slow, writhing movements, usually of all limbs, although the arms are usually more affected than the legs. Other movements that are noted include chorea (rapid, jerky movements), dystonia (fixed postures), ballismus (wide amplitude flailing movements), and tremor (small amplitude, distal movements). The predominant gaze abnormality seen in kernicterus is an upward gaze. The most common auditory disturbance noted is a high-frequency hearing loss.

Incidence

Kernicterus is not a reportable condition in the United States, so its actual prevalence is unknown. In the mid-1900s, kernicterus was a common complication of hyperbilirubinemia associated with hemolytic disease, namely Rh isoimmunization. Kernicterus appeared less often after the introduction of exchange transfusions for hemolytic disease. In 1968, Rh immunoglobulin (RhoGAM) was introduced and all but eliminated erythroblastosis fetalis.[5] By the 1970s, phototherapy had drastically reduced the need for exchange transfusion and kernicterus virtually disappeared in full-term infants.[47]

In the shoulder years of the millennia, several reports documented the association of kernicterus with high serum bilirubin levels.[51,72–74] International case reports came from Europe,[74,75] Africa,[76] the Middle and Far East,[77,78] and New Zealand.[79] Most of these cases did not have obvious hemolytic disease or other recognized cause of neonatal jaundice. Many were healthy breastfeeding newborns, and a large percentage was born at less than 38 weeks' gestation. In response to published reports of kernicterus in otherwise healthy babies, Johnson and associates began a registry for full-term and near-term infants in 1992. They documented 90 cases of kernicterus in 21 states from 1984 to 2001.[51]

Why the Increase

Increased reports of kernicterus occurred temporally in association with significant changes in maternal breastfeeding habits and health care practices. This relationship may serve as the basis for understanding the causes of the resurgence of kernicterus.[80] A significant change in health care practices in the 1990s was the shortening of hospital stays.[81] The impact of early discharge was twofold. First, in full-term newborns, TSB levels do not peak until 48 to 72 hours. Discharge before 48 hours means that peak bilirubin levels do not occur until the newborn is at home. The major increase in milk volume of breastfeeding mothers does not emerge until after 2 or 3 days postpartum. Early discharge increases the risk of inadequate fluid and nutrition intake in these newborns, especially infants less than 38 weeks' gestation. The second change that occurred in association with the rise in kernicterus was the rise of breastfeeding rates. In the 1960s, 30% of mothers were breastfeeding at discharge, compared with 65% in 2001.[82] Many of the kernicterus cases in the recent years involved babies who were breastfed.[73]

A concern over the increased number of reported cases prompted three national agencies to publish alerts for the health care community in 2001. The Joint Commission issued a Sentinel Event Alert,[7] which called for health care organizations to take steps to raise awareness among neonatal caregivers of the potential for kernicterus and its risk factors. The AAP was concomitantly in the process of revising the 1994 practice parameter (guidelines) on hyperbilirubinemia and published a commentary[83] reiterating risk factors for severe hyperbilirubinemia, describing potentially correctable causes of kernicterus, and re-emphasizing the need to evaluate infants jaundiced in the first 24 hours of life for possible hemolytic disease and the importance of follow-up for all newborns discharged at less than 48 hours of age. The revised AAP guidelines were subsequently published in 2004.[6] In the *Morbidity and Mortality Weekly Report*,[47] the Centers for Disease Control and Prevention emphasized the need for early detection of hyperbilirubinemia to prevent the irreversible effects of kernicterus.

Bilirubin-Induced Neuronal Injury in Premature Infants

Premature infants are considered to be at greater risk for developing kernicterus than full-term infants.[84–87] Kernicterus has occurred in low birth weight premature infants with peak TSB levels as low as 6.5 mg/dL.[88] Attempts to find a causal relationship between a specific TSB level and kernicterus, however, have been elusive. Although kernicterus is considered a rare event in the neonatal intensive care unit, reviews of the recent kernicterus cases have identified the late preterm gestation (34 0/7–36 6/7) as a significant risk factor for the development of severe hyperbilirubinemia.[7] Unlike very low birth weight infants who are cared for in neonatal intensive care units, late preterm infants are often cared for in normal newborn nurseries, where caretakers may treat them as full-term infants.[1] Late preterm infants deserve the same vigilance in regards to assessment and management of hyperbilirubinemia as all preterm infants.

ASSESSMENT, SCREENING, AND DIAGNOSIS
Visual Assessment of Jaundice

All infants should be assessed routinely for the development of jaundice.[6] Assessing for jaundice should be performed in a well-lit room and is best performed by blanching the skin with slight finger pressure and noting the underlying color of the skin and subcutaneous tissue. Jaundice is usually visible when bilirubin levels are 5 to 7 mg/dL, appearing first on the face and progressing caudally to the trunk and extremities.[12,89] Although bilirubin levels associated with the progression of jaundice have been described,[89] reliance on visual assessment of jaundice as an estimate of serum bilirubin has been shown to be unreliable[90,91] and is discouraged.[6,11]

Laboratory Evaluation

A key element of the current AAP guidelines requires that measurement of TSB or TcB levels be performed on any infant who is jaundiced in the first 24 hours of life. **Table 1** provides further details for laboratory studies that should be performed on jaundiced infants.

Total serum bilirubin
Measurement of TSB level is one of the most commonly performed laboratory tests performed in newborns.[9] Although the ability to accurately and precisely quantify the various bilirubin fractions in serum or plasma has been—and continues to be—challenging and fraught with inaccuracies, TSB remains the gold standard for diagnosing and treating hyperbilirubinemia in newborns, particularly in the subset of newborns for whom TcB has not been established (see later discussion).[92–96]

Table 1
Laboratory evaluation of the jaundiced infant of 35 or more weeks' gestation

Indications	Assessments
Jaundice in first 24 h	Measure TcB and/or TSB
Jaundice appears excessive for infant's age	Measure TcB and/or TSB
Infant receiving phototherapy or TSB rising rapidly (ie, crossing percentiles [see **Fig. 3**]) and unexplained by history and physical examination	Blood type and Coombs' test, if not obtained with cord blood Complete blood count and smear Measure direct or conjugated bilirubin It is an option to perform reticulocyte count, G6PD, and ETCO$_c$, if available Repeat TSB in 4–24 h depending on infant's age and TSB level
TSB concentration approaching exchange levels or not responding to phototherapy	Perform reticulocyte count, G6PD, albumin, ETCO$_c$, if available
Elevated direct (or conjugated) bilirubin level	Do urinalysis and urine culture; evaluate for sepsis if indicated by history and physical examination
Jaundice present at or beyond age 3 wk or sick infant	Total and direct (or conjugated) bilirubin level If direct bilirubin elevated, evaluate for causes of cholestasis Check results of newborn thyroid and galactosemia screen and evaluate infant for signs or symptoms of hypothyroidism

From American Academy of Pediatrics Subcommittee on Hyperbilirubinemia. Management of hyperbilirubinemia in the newborn infant 35 or more weeks of gestation. Pediatrics 2004;114:300; with permission.

Several fractions of bilirubin exist in the blood, yet traditional measurement methods do not quantify each fraction separately. The terms "direct" and "indirect" refer to the way bilirubin reacts to a dye known as diazotized sulfanilic acid. Conjugated and delta bilirubin (unconjugated bilirubin bound covalently to albumin) react directly with the diazo agent and are reported as direct bilirubin. Unconjugated bilirubin (free and bound with albumin fractions) reacts only when an accelerant is added to the mixture and is reported as indirect bilirubin. The terms direct and indirect have been used interchangeably with conjugated and unconjugated, respectively, but this is not quantitatively correct because the measurement of direct bilirubin includes delta bilirubin.[97] This practice has little clinical relevance because levels of delta bilirubin are insignificant in newborns. Traditional measurements for bilirubin report the total and direct bilirubin values. Indirect bilirubin concentrations are derived from the total bilirubin concentration minus the direct bilirubin concentration.

Two studies that compared TSB measurements from capillary and venous samples provided conflicting results.[98,99] Maisels[9] pointed out that the published data on the relationship between TSB levels and kernicterus are based on capillary samples, however. The AAP[6] recommends against obtaining a venous sample to confirm capillary results because it delays the initiation of treatment.

Bilirubin/albumin ratio and free bilirubin
The ratio of TSB to albumin has been shown to correlate with unbound bilirubin and can be used as a proxy for the measurement of unbound bilirubin.[100] The B/A ratio is a factor that can be considered in the decision to initiate phototherapy or perform exchange transfusion.[6] Evaluation of the B/A ratio must be made in context of understanding that albumin levels and albumin binding capacity vary significantly among newborns. Although the B/A ratio may be used when evaluating jaundiced infants, it must be used in conjunction with TSB levels when making a decision regarding the need for an exchange transfusion.[6] Several authors advocated that the measurement of free bilirubin is a more useful predictor of brain toxicity than TSB.[101–103] Because free bilirubin is the fraction that crosses the blood-brain barrier, this argument makes sense theoretically.

Widespread use of free bilirubin measurement is limited by the lack of instruments that can accurately and unequivocally measure free bilirubin. Acceptance of free bilirubin as a better predictor is hindered by a lack of scientific evidence that clearly establishes the clinical meaning of values.[104,105]

The National Institute of Child Health and Human Development[106] recognized the existence of a knowledge and service gap in the assessment and measurement of bilirubin levels, particularly as they relate to bilirubin-induced brain injury and kernicterus. The institute has called for the validation of effective methods for evaluation of B/A binding and free bilirubin. Also essential for narrowing the service gap is implementation of regulatory standards to improve interlaboratory consistency and reliability for bilirubin measurement and evaluation.

Transcutaneous Bilirubinometry

Noninvasive TcB measurements have become a valued tool in the screening of term and near-term infants for hyperbilirubinemia.[6,65,107] The Bili-Check (Respironics, Norcross, GA) and Jaundice Meter JM-103 (Konica Minolta Sensing, Osaka, Japan) are the two devices available in the United States. Numerous studies have validated the accuracy of these instruments in multiracial populations and term and near-term newborn infants, generally proving values within 2 to 3 mg/dL of the TSB if the TSB level is less than 15 mg/dL.[34,107–114]

Several studies have demonstrated clinical accuracy of the BiliCheck in racially diverse populations.[108,111,114] Engle and associates[115] found that the device underestimated TSB levels in a Hispanic population of newborns at 35 or more weeks' gestation. The BiliCheck instrument transmits white light into the skin of the newborn and collects and analyzes the reflected light. Because the characteristics of skin and underlying tissues that affect spectral reflectance are known, spectral subtraction can be used to derive the bilirubin concentration.[115] The JM-102, predecessor of the Jaundice Meter JM-103, performed less well in black infants. The newer JM-103 determines yellowness of subcutaneous tissue by using two optical paths to measure optical density difference at two wavelengths. With the use of a short and long optical path, light returning to the sensor from shallow tissue, such as the dermis, is separated from light returning from the subcutaneous tissue.[116] This difference allows evaluation of bilirubin levels in the subcutaneous tissue without the influence of skin pigmentation. In a study of 849 newborns aged 35 weeks' gestation or older,

Maisels and Ostrea[113] demonstrated accuracy of the JM-103 in a multiracial population that included white, black, east Asian, Indian/Pakistani, and Hispanic infants. The correlation of TcB and TSB was less close in the black infants more often than in other groups, with the TcB overestimating bilirubin levels. The differences between TcB and TSB grew as serum bilirubin levels increased. The authors concluded, however, that the JM-103 is clinically acceptable because it overestimated serum bilirubin levels, and decisions based on TcB levels would not be clinically dangerous.

Several limitations to transcutaneous bilirubinometry still exist. There is a paucity of data on the accuracy of TcB measurements when TSB levels are 15 mg/dL or more; as such, they should be used with caution when TcB values are approximating 15 mg/dL. The accuracy of transcutaneous bilirubin instruments in low birth weight infants, newborns younger than 35 weeks' gestation, or infants receiving phototherapy has yet to be established.

ETCOc

When heme oxygenase breaks down heme, equimolar quantities of CO and biliverdin are produced. Biliverdin is rapidly reduced to bilirubin, and CO binds with hemoglobin to be eliminated from the body by the lungs. The measurement of CO in the end-tidal breath, corrected for ambient CO (ETCOc), is a useful index of bilirubin production and hemolysis. Measurement of ETCOc has been shown to aid in the differentiation between infants with and without hemolysis and the identification of infants with impaired conjugation defects who have a normal ETCOc level with rising TSB levels.[117] The AAP[6] includes ETCOc as an assessment tool to be used when (1) TSB concentrations are approaching exchange levels or not responding to phototherapy or (2) for infants receiving phototherapy or when TSB is rising rapidly and is unexplained by history and physical examination (**Table 1**).

RISK PREDICTION

Before discharge, every newborn should be assessed for the risk of developing severe hyperbilirubinemia.[6] Risk assessment is performed using two methods, used individually or in combination. The best method of assessing risk of subsequent hyperbilirubinemia is done by measuring the TSB or TcB level and plotting the value on an hour-specific nomogram that identifies risk levels (**Fig. 3**). Alternatively, or in combination, the clinician can evaluate the infant for the presence of risk factors. Risk factors commonly associated with an increase risk of severe hyperbilirubinemia are contained in **Box 1**.[6] The risk factors most frequently associated with severe hyperbilirubinemia are breastfeeding, gestation less than 38 weeks, significant jaundice in a previous sibling, and jaundice noted before discharge.[6,118,119]

Recently, Keren and colleagues[120] compared the predictive ability of the risk assessment strategies individually and in combination. They found that the only clinical risk factor that improved

---

Box 1
Risk factors for severe hyperbilirubinemia

Major risk factors

  Predischarge TSB or TcB level in the high-risk zone (**Fig. 3**)

  Jaundice observed in the first 24 hours

  Blood group incompatibility with positive direct antiglobulin test, other known hemolytic disease (eg, G6PD deficiency), elevated ETCO$_c$

  Gestational age 35–36 weeks

  Previous sibling having received phototherapy

  Cephalohematoma or significant bruising

  Exclusive breastfeeding, particularly if nursing is not going well and weight loss is excessive

  East Asian race

Minor risk factors

  Predischarge TSB or TcB level in the high intermediate-risk zone

  Gestational age 37–38 weeks

  Jaundice observed before discharge

  Previous sibling with jaundice

  Macrosomic infant of a mother who has diabetes

  Maternal age 25 years

  Male gender

Decreased risk (these factors associated with decreased risk of significant jaundice, listed in order of decreasing importance)

  TSB or TcB level in the low-risk zone (**Fig. 3**)

  Gestational age 41 weeks

  Exclusive bottle feeding

  Black race

  Discharge from hospital after 72 hours

overall accuracy of the predischarge risk zone was gestational age. They concluded that two things—gestational age and predischarge bililirubin level— are accurate predictors of or risks for developing significant hyperbilirubinemia. Their work may pave the way for future recommendations on risk assessment.

TREATMENT
Phototherapy

Introduced in 1958 by Cremer and colleagues,[121] phototherapy is the most common treatment modality currently used in the management of hyperbilirubinemia.[4] Phototherapy is used to prevent TSB levels from reaching a level at which exchange transfusion is recommended.[6] Guidelines for phototherapy in infants at 35 or more weeks' gestation have been identified by the AAP (**Fig. 4**). Defining guidelines for phothotherapy in infants younger than 35 weeks has proved elusive. The aim of reducing bilirubin is to prevent injury that can lead to kernicterus or other developmental disability. Because it has not been possible to relate specific TSB levels in low birth weight infants to these outcomes, it has been difficult to assign evidence-based specific bilirubin levels at which phototherapy or exchange transfusion should be initiated in low birth weight infants. **Tables 2** and **3** provide guidance for clinicians and reflect the opinions of experts.

An additional goal of treatment is to not cause harm. There is growing concern that decreasing bilirubin levels may confiscate the powerful antioxidant effects of bilirubin in a population that is already antioxidant deficient.[6] The National Institute of Child Health and Human Development Neonatal Research Network is currently conducting a prospective randomized trial to compare aggressive to conservative phototherapy in low birth weight infants. The study focuses on neurodevelopmental impairment outcome at 18 to 22 months or death and should provide important information about the use of phototherapy in low birth weight infants.

How it works
Phototherapy uses light energy directed at the skin to change the shape and structure of bilirubin molecules residing in the skin and subcutaneous tissue into molecules that can be excreted without undergoing conjugation by the liver. The rate of reduction of serum bilirubin concentrations depends on the rate of bilirubin photoalteration, the transport of the photoproducts (products of photoalteration), and elimination of these

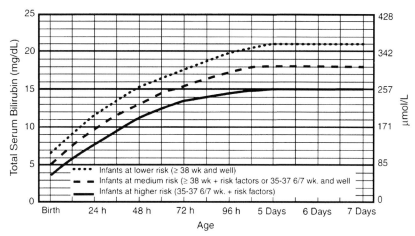

Fig. 4. Guidelines for phototherapy in hospitalized infants of 35 or more weeks' gestation. Use total bilirubin. Do not subtract direct reacting or conjugated bilirubin. Risk factors = isoimmune hemolytic disease, G6PD deficiency, asphyxia, significant lethargy, temperature instability, sepsis, acidosis, or albumin < 3.0 g/dL (if measured). For well infants aged 35–37 weeks' gestation, can adjust TSB levels for intervention around the medium risk line. It is an option to intervene at lower TSB levels for infants closer to 35 weeks and at higher TSB levels for infant closer to 37 6/7 weeks. It is an option to provide conventional phototherapy in hospital or at home at TSB levels 2–3 mg/dL (35–50 mmol/L) below those shown, but home phototherapy should not be used in any infant with risk factors. Note: These guidelines are based on limited evidence and the levels shown are approximations. The guidelines refer to the use of intensive phototherapy, which should be used when the TSB exceeds the line indicated for each category. Infants are designated as "higher risk" because of the potential negative effects of the conditions listed on albumin binding of bilirubin, the blood-brain barrier, and the susceptibility of the brain cells to damage by bilirubin. "Intensive phototherapy" implies irradiance in the blue-green spectrum (wavelengths of approximately 430–490 nm) of at least 30 µW/cm²/nm (measured at the infant's skin directly below the center of the phototherapy unit) and delivered to as much of the infant's surface area as possible. Note that irradiance measured below the center of the light source is much greater than that measured at the periphery. Measurements should be made with a radiometer specified by the manufacturer of the phototherapy system. If TSB levels approach or exceed the exchange transfusion line (see **Fig. 6**), the sides of the bassinet, incubator, or warmer should be lined with aluminum foil or white material, which increases the surface area of the infant exposed and increases the efficacy of phototherapy. If the TSB level does not decrease or continues to rise in an infant who is receiving intensive phototherapy, this strongly suggests the presence of hemolysis. Infants who receive phototherapy and have an elevated direct-reacting or conjugated bilirubin level (cholestatic jaundice) may develop the bronze-baby syndrome. (*From* American Academy of Pediatrics Subcommittee on Hyperbilirubinemia. Management of hyperbilirubinemia in the newborn infant 35 or more weeks of gestation. Pediatrics 2004;114(1):304; with permission.)

products. It is believed that photoalteration is the rate-limiting step.[4]

When bilirubin absorbs light within its absorption spectrum, the molecule enters a transient excited state that can react with oxygen to form colorless polar molecules (photo-oxidation products) that can be excreted in the urine.[2,4] Photo-oxidation accounts for only a small portion of bilirubin reduction by phototherapy.[4] Bilirubin molecules that do not undergo photo-oxidation can undergo rearrangement to become isomers of the native bilirubin molecule. Configurational isomerization produces bilirubin molecules that are more water soluble and less toxic. Configurational isomerization is a reversible process, however, and these molecules can revert to the more native and lipid-soluble molecule. Structural isomerization is

an irreversible alteration to the bilirubin molecule that forms lumirubin, another water-soluble product that can be excreted in the bile and urine. **Fig. 5** illustrates the mechanism of phototherapy.

Factors that determine effectiveness
Effectiveness of phototherapy is influenced by the spectral qualities of the light source, the delivered spectral irradiance, and the amount of body surface area exposed to the light source.

Spectral qualities
In order for phototherapy to work, bilirubin must absorb a particle of light, referred to as a photon. Only light of certain colors (or wavelengths) can be absorbed by bilirubin. To be absorbed by bilirubin, the photon must have a wavelength that

Table 2
Guidelines for the use of phototherapy and exchange transfusion in low-birth-weight infants based on birth weight

Birth weight (g)	Total Bilirubin Level (mg/dL [μmol/L])[a]	
	Phototherapy[b]	Exchange Transfusion[c]
≤1500	5–8 (85–140)	13–16 (220–275)
1500–1999	8–12 (140–200)	16–18 (275–300)
2000–2499	11–14 (190–240)	18–20 (300–340)

Note that these guidelines reflect ranges used in neonatal intensive care units. They cannot take into account all possible situations. Lower bilirubin concentrations should be used for infants who are sick (eg, sepsis, acidosis, hypoalbuminemia) or who have hemolytic disease.

[a] Consider initiating therapy at these levels. Range allows discretion based on clinical conditions or other circumstances. Note that bilirubin levels refer to TSB concentrations. Direct-reacting or conjugated levels should not be subtracted from the total.

[b] Used at these levels and in therapeutic doses, phototherapy should, with few exceptions, eliminate the need for exchange transfusions.

[c] Levels for exchange transfusion assume that bilirubin continues to rise or remains at these levels despite intensive phototherapy.

Adapted from Maisels MJ. Jaundice. In: MacDonald MG, Mullett MD, Seshia MMK, editors. Avery's neonatology: pathophysiology & management of the newborn. 6th edition. Philadelphia: Lippincott Williams & Wilkins; 2005. p. 818; with permission.

matches the bilirubin absorption spectrum. Because bilirubin has a yellow color, it can absorb only violet, blue, or green light. Bilirubin absorbs light best that has a wavelength near 460 nm, which is in the blue spectrum.[2] Wavelengths of light must penetrate the skin to reach the bilirubin molecule and have any effect. Because the transmittance of light through the skin increases with increasing wavelength, Maisels[2] suggested that the best wavelengths to use for phototherapy when treating hyperbilirubinemia are in the blue-green spectrum with a range of 460 to 490 nm.

The spectrum of light delivered is determined by the type of light source and any filters used. Light sources used in phototherapy include fluorescent tubes, tungsten, halogen, light-emitting diodes, and fiberoptic lights, all of which are effective for standard phototherapy. When TSB concentrations approach the level at which intensive phototherapy is required, however, only those that deliver light in the blue-green spectrum should be used.[6] "Special blue" fluorescent lamps are the most effective because they provide light primarily in that spectrum. Recently, light-emitting diode lights have been found to be as effective as "special blue" fluorescent lamps.[122]

Irradiance

Irradiance refers to light intensity and represents the number of photons delivered per square centimeter of the exposed body surface area.[4] Irradiance is also referred to as spectral irradiance and is expressed as $\mu W/cm^2/nm$. Irradiance can be thought of as dose. The higher the irradiance, the higher the dose and the faster bilirubin declines.[123] The spectral irradiance of each type

Table 3
Guidelines for use of phototherapy and exchange transfusion in preterm infants based on gestational age

Gestational Age (wk)	Total Bilirubin Level (mg/dL [μmol/L])		
	Phototherapy	Exchange Transfusion	
		Sick[a]	Well
36	14.6 (250)	17.5 (300)	20.5 (350)
32	8.8 (150)	14.6 (250)	17.5 (300)
28	5.8 (100)	11.7 (200)	14.6 (250)
24	4.7 (80)	8.8 (150)	11.7 (200)

[a] Rhesus disease, perinatal asphyxia, hypoxia, acidosis, hypercapnia.

From Ives NK. Neonatal jaundice. In: Rennie JM, editor. Robertson's textbook of neonatology. 4th edition. Philadelphia: Elsevier Churchill Livingstone; 2005. p. 675; with permission.

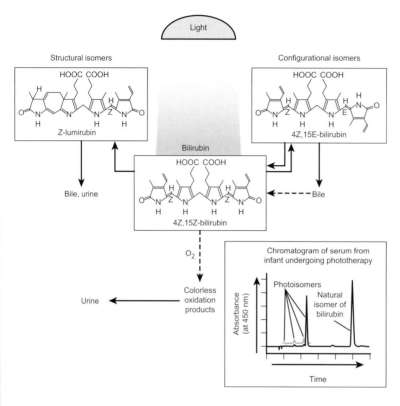

Fig. 5. Mechanism of photo-therapy. The absorption of light by the normal form of bilirubin (4Z,15Z-bilirubin) generates transient excited-state bilirubin molecules. These fleeting intermediates can react with oxygen to produce colorless products of lower molecular weight or they can undergo rearrangement to become structural isomers (lumirubins) or isomers in which the configuration of at least one of the two Z-configuration double bonds has changed to an E configuration. (Z and E, from the German *zusammen* [together] and *entgegen* [opposite] are prefixes used for designating the stereochemistry around a double bond. The prefixes 4 and 15 designate double-bond positions.) Only the two principal photoisomers formed in humans are shown. Configurational isomerization is reversible and much faster than structural isomerization, which is irreversible. Both occur much more quickly than photo-oxidation. The photoisomers are less lipophilic than the 4Z,15Z form of bilirubin and can be excreted unchanged in bile without undergoing glucuronidation. Lumirubin isomers can also be excreted in urine. Photo-oxidation products are excreted mainly in urine. Once in bile, configurational isomers revert spontaneously to the natural 4Z,15Z form of bilirubin. The graph, a high-performance liquid chromatogram of serum from an infant undergoing phototherapy, shows the presence of several photoisomers in addition to the 4Z,15Z isomer. Photoisomers are also detectable in the blood of healthy adults after sunbathing. (*From* Maisels MJ, McDonagh AF. Phototherapy for neonatal jaundice. N Engl J Med 2008;358:922; with permission.)

of light source is different, and the delivered spectral irradiance depends on the distance between the light source and the infant. Traditional daylight phototherapy delivers a spectral irradiance of 8 to 10 μW/cm^2/nm, which is acceptable for standard phototherapy.[6] Conversely, intensive phototherapy requires spectral irradiance more than 30 μW/cm^2/nm.

The greater the distance between the light source and the infant's skin, the less the delivered spectral irradiance. The easiest solution to increase delivered spectral irradiance of a phototherapy unit is to move it closer to the infant. Halogen spot lights must not be positioned closer to the infant than the manufacturer recommends because halogen lights can generate significant amounts of heat and cause thermal injury to the infant. When treating term and late preterm infants, the AAP[6] recommends placing the infant in a bassinet or open crib and positioning the light source 10 to 15 cm above the infant. Special

blue tubes positioned as such produce an irradiance of at least 35 μW/cm^2/nm.

Radiometers ("bili meters") are used to measure spectral irradiance within a specified wavelength. Most radiometers are designed by a manufacturer to be used with its light source and can produce significantly inaccurate results if used to measure irradiance of a different manufacturer's product.[4] When measuring spectral irradiance, clinicians should use the device recommended by the manufacturer of the phototherapy unit. Measured irradiance is also affected by where the measurement is taken. When measured below the center of the light source, irradiance can be twice that measured at the periphery.[2,6] Ideally, several measurements of irradiance should be obtained at several sites under the light source and the measurements averaged.[6] If this is not possible, measuring irradiance below the center of the lights is acceptable.[2] Although measurement of irradiance is not necessary before each use of a phototherapy unit, periodic checks of irradiance should be performed.[6]

Body surface area

Tan[124] demonstrated that the greater the amount of body surface area exposed to phototherapy, the greater the decline in bilirubin levels. Maximizing exposed body surface area is done by providing phototherapy from above and below infants. The BiliBlanket (Olympic Medical, Seattle, WA) is a commercially available unit that does this. Placing fiberoptic pads below an infant and lamps above accomplishes the same goal. In low birth weight infants, this method is twice as effective as conventional phototherapy alone[125,126] but only 50% more effective than single phototherapy in full-term infants.[126] The difference in response is possibly related to the size of the fiberoptic pads in relation to the size of the infant. Full-term infants with high bilirubin levels may require two or three pads underneath them.[127]

Delivery systems

Various delivery systems are available to provide phototherapy to infants. Traditional phototherapy has been administered via fluorescent bulbs. Bulbs used in these systems include daylight, white, blue, "special blue," or a combination of these.[128] Not all fluorescent bulbs are the same, however. The bulbs with the greatest irradiance—and the most effective—are the "special blue" tubes. These bulbs carry the label F20T12/BB (General Electric Westinghouse, Sylvania). Regular fluorescent bulbs are labeled F20T12/B. Halogen lights cast a spot of light that has a high irradiance only in the center. Toward the periphery of the spot, irradiance has been reported as low as 7 $\mu W/cm^2/nm$.[4] More than one spotlight may be required to deliver sufficient irradiance to the entire exposed surface area of infants, particularly full-term infants. Halogen spotlights are convenient but can generate a considerable amount of heat. Fiberoptic blankets incorporate a quartz-halogen bulb housed inside a light box that delivers light through a fiberoptic cable to a pad, which is placed under the infant. The main advantage of this system is that infants can be held without interrupting phototherapy.

A Cochrane review[129] concluded that single fiberoptic phototherapy was less effective than conventional phototherapy. When two fiberoptic devices were used, this method was equally effective as conventional phototherapy in preterm infants. A combination of fiberoptic and conventional phototherapy was more effective than conventional phototherapy alone. The newest phototherapy system available uses high-intensity gallium nitride light emitting diodes (neoBLUE, Natus Medical, Inc., San Carlos, CA) and delivers light in the blue to blue-green spectrum. Light-emitting diode units are effective and able to provide intensive phototherapy, generating irradiance of at least 30 $\mu W/cm^2/nm$.[6] Light-emitting diode units also have the advantages of being efficient, generating little heat, and lasting much longer.[4] For a more thorough discussion of phototherapy delivery systems, the reader is directed to recent reviews.[4,128]

Side effects

Serious adverse effects of phototherapy are rare.[2] Bronze baby syndrome, a condition in which the skin, serum, and urine develop a dark, grayish-brown discoloration, occurs only in infants with unconjugated hyperbilirubinemia. The pathogenesis of this condition is not fully understood but may be related to an accumulation of porphyrins and other metabolites.[9] Not all cholestatic infants treated with phototherapy develop bronze baby syndrome. Purpuric and bullous eruptions also have been reported in cholestatic infants who received phototherapy. Infants with congenital erythropoietic porphyria or who are receiving photosensitization agents have been reported to develop severe blistering and photosensitivity during phototherapy.[130,131] These conditions are absolute contraindications to phototherapy.[2,6]

Conventional phototherapy can cause changes to the thermal environment and result in thermal instability and increased insensible water loss.[132,133] When conventional phototherapy is initiated for an infant being cared for in an air-controlled environment, close attention should be paid to the infant's temperature, which can rise rapidly and require a decrease in the environmental set point.[128] When phototherapy is discontinued under the same condition, the environmental temperature may need to be increased. When skin servocontrol is used, there is a decrease in air temperature after initiation of phototherapy because conventional phototherapy warms the infant.[133] Dollberg and colleagues[133] demonstrated fluctuations in air temperature for 3 hours before reaching steady state. Changes to the thermal environment when light-emitting diode lights are used have not been investigated thoroughly.

Insensible water loss occurs as a result of increased peripheral blood flow and has been shown to occur with conventional fluorescent bulbs and halogen spotlights. Grunhagen and colleagues[134] demonstrated that transepidermal water loss increased approximately 20% in preterm infants receiving phototherapy using halogen spotlights despite constant skin temperature and relative humidity of 52%. Maayan-Metger and colleagues[135] found similar results in preterm infants receiving phototherapy using fluorescent lamps. Monitoring urine output, urine specific gravity, serum electrolytes, and changes in weight is an important nursing consideration when caring for infants receiving phototherapy.

A recent concern was introduced by Csoma and associates,[136,137] who reported an increased incidence of dysplastic nevi in children who received blue light phototherapy as infants. More research is needed on this topic because dysplastic nevi increase the risk for the development of malignant melanoma. Light can cause injury to the retina, and infants must have their eyes covered with opaque patches. Additional side effects of phototherapy include loose bowel movements, temporary lactose intolerance, decreased platelet count, potential interference with circadian rhythm, and potential interference with parent-infant bonding.[46]

Monitoring effectiveness of phototherapy

The goal of phototherapy is to decrease circulating bilirubin and prevent it from increasing.[2] Bilirubin levels decline most quickly in the first 4 to 6 hours of phototherapy.[6] A decrease in bilirubin levels of 6% to 20% of initial levels can be expected in the first 24 hours of standard phototherapy.[126,138] The rate of decline in bilirubin levels depends not only on light dose but also on the cause and severity of hyperbilirubinemia. Combination or double phototherapy can increase the rate of bilirubin reduction, primarily by increasing the amount of surface area exposed to the light. Bilirubin levels do not decline as rapidly during active hemolysis as they would without hemolysis. When bilirubin levels are high and there is more bilirubin in the subcutaneous tissues, phototherapy produces rapid declines in TSB levels. Intensive phototherapy can decrease TSB levels by as much as 10 mg/dL within 5 hours when TSB levels are more than 30 mg/dL[139] and drop by 30% to 40% within 24 hours.[140] When phototherapy is discontinued, one can expect a rebound increase in TSB levels of 1 to 2 mg/dL.[140] Infants at risk for significant increases in TSB after discontinuation of phototherapy are preterm, have hemolytic disease, or were treated with phototherapy before 72 hours of age.[2,141]

Exchange Transfusion

Before the discovery of phototherapy, exchange transfusion was the treatment required to reduce serum bilirubin levels and prevent kernicterus. Over time, the performance of exchange transfusion has decreased in frequency and is an unusual occurrence in neonatal intensive care units.[142,143] Guidelines for exchange transfusion in infants 35 or more weeks' gestation are identified in **Fig. 6**. See **Tables 2** and **3** for similar guidelines for low birth weight infants.

During an exchange transfusion, twice the infant's blood volume (170 mL/kg) is exchanged in small aliquots (not to exceed 10% of the total blood volume) and replaced with equal aliquots of donor blood, usually packed RBCs reconstituted with plasma. The procedure is usually performed through two central catheters. The double volume exchange transfusion replaces approximately 85% of the infant's blood volume and reduces bilirubin levels by approximately 40% at the end of the procedure.[10,31] Serum bilirubin levels can rise to 70% to 80% of pre-exchange levels within 30 minutes of the procedure because of re-equilibration that occurs between the vascular and extravascular compartment.[31] When the procedure is performed on an infant with immune-mediated hemolytic disease, it has the added benefit of removing antibody-coated RBCs and maternal antibody and correcting anemia. The AAP[6] recommends the administration of intravenous gamma globulin (0.5–1 g/kg over 2 hours) for infants with isoimmune hemolytic disease if the TSB level is rising despite intensive phototherapy or the TSB level is within 2 to 3 mg/dL of the exchange level.

Potential complications of exchange transfusion include thrombocytopenia (especially with repeat transfusions), hypocalcemia, hypomagnesemia, hypoglycemia, arrhythmia, cardiac arrest, respiratory or metabolic acidosis, rebound metabolic alkalosis, and complications associated with blood transfusion and umbilical vessel catheterization. The exchange transfusion–related mortality rate has been reported as 0.1% to 0.5%. Because exchange transfusions are performed much less frequently, previously reported rates for morbidity and mortality may not apply.[6,10] To study this concern, Steiner and colleagues[142] performed a retrospective review of 107 patients who received 141 exchange transfusions between 1986 and 1996. Despite the decline in the number of exchange transfusions performed over time, they did not find a significant difference in transfusion-related complications in the eras before and after the 1994 AAP practice guideline on the management of hyperbilirubinemia.

Drug Therapy

Phenobarbital

Phenobarbital enhances conjugation of bilirubin in the liver by inducing glucuronyl transferase

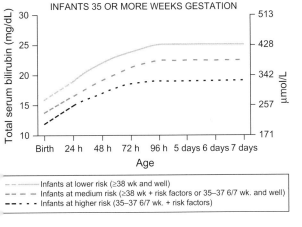

GUIDELINES FOR EXCHANGE TRANSFUSION IN INFANTS 35 OR MORE WEEKS GESTATION

- - - Infants at lower risk (≥38 wk and well)
- - - Infants at medium risk (≥38 wk + risk factors or 35–37 6/7 wk. and well)
- - - Infants at higher risk (35–37 6/7 wk. + risk factors)

Fig. 6. Guidelines for exchange transfusion in infants 35 or more weeks' gestation. The dashed lines for the first 24 hours indicate uncertainity due to a wide range of clinical circumstances and a range of responses to phototherapy. Immediate exchange transfusion is recommended if an infant shows signs of acute bilirubin encephalopathy (hypertonia, arching, retrocollis, opisthotonos, fever, high-pitched cry) or if TSB is ≥ 5mg/dL (85 μmol/L) above these lines. Risk factors include isoimmune hemolytic disease, G6PD deficiency, asphyxia, significant lethargy, temperature instability, sepsis, and acidosis. Measure serum albumin and calculate B/A ratio (see legend). Use total bilirubin. Do not subtract direct reacting or conjugated bilirubin. If infant is well and 35–37 weeks' gestation (median risk), you can individualize TSB levels for exchange based on actual gestational age. Note that these suggested levels represent a consensus of most of the committee but are based on limited evidence, and the levels shown are approximations. (See the article by Bhutani VK[3] for risks and complications of exchange transfusion.) During birth hospitalization, exchange transfusion is recommended if the TSB rises to these levels despite intensive phototherapy. For readmitted infants, if the TSB level is above the exchange level, repeat TSB measurement every 2 to 3 hours and consider exchange if the TSB remains above the levels indicated after intensive phototherapy for 6 hours. If the TSB is at or approaching the exchange level, send blood for immediate type and cross-match. Blood for exchange transfusion is modified whole blood (red cells and plasma) cross-matched against the mother and compatible with the infant. (*From* American Academy of Pediatrics Subcommittee on Hyperbilirubinemia. Management of hyperbilirubinemia in the newborn infant 35 or more weeks of gestation. Pediatrics. 2004;114(1):305; with permission.) The following B/A ratios can be used together with but not in lieu of the TSB level as an additional factor in determining the need for exchange transfusion:

Risk Category	B/A Ratio at Which Exchange Transfusion Should be Considered	
	TSB mg/dL/Alb, g/dL	TSB μmol/L/Alb, μmol/L
Infants ≥ 38 0/7 wk	8.0	0.94
Infants 35 0/7–36 6/7 wk and well or ≥ 38 0/7 wk if higher risk or isoimmune hemolytic disease or G6PD deficiency	7.2	0.84
Infants 35 0/7–37 6/7 wk if higher risk or isoimmune hemolytic disease or G6PD deficiency	6.8	0.8

activity. Phenobarbital also increases bile flow, but its effect takes a few days, which is an undesirable characteristic for the management of acute hyperbilirubinemia.

Intravenous immunoglobulin

The administration of intravenous immunoglobulin to infants with Rh isoimmunization has been shown to decrease the need for exchange transfusion[144–146] and is considered effective for ABO hemolytic disease.[147] A systematic review conducted by Gottstein and Cooke[148] concluded that intravenous immunoglobulin reduced the duration of phototherapy and hospital stay in infants with hemolytic disease. The mechanism of action is not thoroughly known, but it is thought that intravenous immunoglobulin may block receptors (Fc receptors) in the reticuloendothelial system that bind to the antibodies that cause cell death and hemolysis.[147,148]

Metalloporphyrins

Most therapies in the armament against hyperbilirubinemia attempt to decrease serum bilirubin levels by increasing the elimination of bilirubin. One novel approach attempts to reduce bilirubin levels by reducing bilirubin production. The rate-limiting enzyme in the conversion of heme to biliverdin is heme oxygenase. Naturally occurring and synthetic metalloporphyrins are powerful competitive inhibitors of heme oxygenase and suppress the formation of bilirubin. Effective metalloporphyrins include zinc, chromium, and manganese, but tin mesoporphyrin has emerged as the preferred agent.[10] When studied in preterm infants, tin mesoporphyrin reduced bilirubin levels by 41% and phototherapy requirements by 76%.[149] In healthy full-term breastfed infants with hyperbilirubinemia, a single dose of tin mesoporphyrin completely eliminated the need for phototherapy.[150] Metalloporphyrins reduce bilirubin levels, but additional studies are needed to evaluate their long-term safety. One tin mesoporphyrin, stannsoporfin (Stanate), is undergoing clinical trials in the United States and is available for compassionate use.

SUMMARY

Hyperbilirubinemia is a ubiquitous phenomenon in newborns. Its existence, not severity, has little regard for birth weight, gestational age, gender, race, or degree of wellness. Usually, hyperbilirubinemia exposes nothing more than the unique aspects of newborn physiology. Origins of a pathologic nature also can manifest with hyperbilirubinemia, and clinicians must know when to investigate for a cause other than maturation. Increased bilirubin levels, no matter the reason, have the potential to cause debilitating, devastating, and irreversible consequences. A plethora of data supports dependable strategies for assessing and managing hyperbilirubinemia in healthy full-term newborns. On the other hand, there is a paucity of equivalent evidence for sick and premature newborns. In the nursery, late preterm infants must be cared for in the context that they are not full term and share similar vulnerabilities as infants of lesser gestational age. In the neonatal intensive care unit, jaundice must not be eclipsed by conditions whose life-threatening consequences are more temporally visible. Clinicians are encouraged to remain attentive to serum bilirubin levels in all infants and respond in accordance with the best evidence currently available.

REFERENCES

1. Watchko JF. Neonatal hyperbilirubinemia: what are the risks? N Engl J Med 2006;354(18):1947–9.
2. Maisels MJ, McDonagh AF. Phototherapy for neonatal jaundice. N Engl J Med 2008;358(9): 920–8.
3. Bhutani VK, Johnson LH, Keren R. Diagnosis and management of hyperbilirubinemia in the term neonate: for a safer first week. Pediatr Clin North Am 2004;51(4):843–61, vii.
4. Vreman HJ, Wong RJ, Stevenson DK. Phototherapy: current methods and future directions. Semin Perinatol 2004;28(5):326–33.
5. American Academy of Pediatrics Provisional Committee for Quality Improvement and Subcommittee on Hyperbilirubinemia. Practice parameter: management of hyperbilirubinemia in the healthy term newborn. Pediatrics 1994;94(4 Pt 1):558–65.
6. American Academy of Pediatrics Subcommittee on Hyperbilirubinemia. Management of hyperbilirubinemia in the newborn infant 35 or more weeks of gestation. Pediatrics 2004;114(1):297–316.
7. The Joint Commission. Kernicterus threatens healthy newborns: sentinel event alert. Available at: http://www.jointcommission.org/SentinelEvents/SentinelEventAlert/sea_18.htm. Accessed June 12, 2008.
8. The Joint Commission. Revised guidance to help prevent kernicterus: sentinel event alert. Available at: http://www.jointcommission.org/SentinelEvents/SentinelEventAlert/sea_31.htm. Accessed June 12, 2008.
9. Maisels MJ. Jaundice. In: MacDonald MG, Mullett MD, Seshia MMK, editors. Avery's neonatology: pathophysiology & management of the newborn. 6th edition. Philadelphia: Lippincott Williams & Wilkins; 2005. p. 768–846.
10. Wong RJ, DeSandre GH, Sibley E, et al. Neonatal jaundice and liver disease. In: Martin RJ, Fanaroff AA, Walsh MC, editors. Fanaroff and Martin's neonatal-perinatal medicine: diseases of the fetus and infant. 8th edition. Philadelphia: Mosby Elsevier; 2006. p. 1419–65.
11. Wong RJ, Stevenson DK, Ahlfors CE, et al. Neonatal jaundice: bilirubin physiology and clinical chemistry. NeoReviews 2007;8:e58–67. Available at: http://neoreviews.aappublications.org/cgi/content/full/neoreviews;8/2/e58. Accessed June 27, 2008.
12. Blackburn ST. Bilirubin metabolism. In: Maternal, fetal, neonatal physiology: a clinical perspective. 2nd edition. St. Louis (MO): WB Saunders; 2003. p. 652–76.
13. Gartner LM. Neonatal jaundice. Pediatr Rev 1994; 15(11):422–32.
14. Bartoletti AL, Stevenson DK, Ostrander CR, et al. Pulmonary excretion of carbon monoxide in the human infant as an index of bilirubin production. I. Effects of gestational and postnatal age and some common neonatal abnormalities. J Pediatr 1979;94(6):952–5.
15. Maisels MJ, Pathak A, Nelson NM, et al. Endogenous production of carbon monoxide in normal and erythroblastic newborn infants. J Clin Invest 1971;50(1):1–8.

16. Maden A, MacMahon JR, Stevenson DK. Neonatal hyperbilirubinemia. In: Taeusch HW, Ballard RA, Gleason CA, editors. Avery's diseases of the newborn. 8th edition. Philadelphia: Elsevier Saunders; 2005. p. 1226–56.

17. Notarianni LJ. Plasma protein binding of drugs in pregnancy and in neonates. Clin Pharm 1990;18(1):20–36.

18. Wolkoff AW, Goresky CA, Sellin J, et al. Role of ligandin in transfer of bilirubin from plasma into liver. Am J Phys 1979;236(6):E638–48.

19. Onishi S, Kawade N, Itoh S, et al. Postnatal development of uridine diphosphate glucuronyltransferase activity towards bilirubin and 2-aminophenol in human liver. Biochem J 1979;184(3):705–7.

20. Kawade N, Onishi S. The prenatal and postnatal development of UDP-glucuronyltransferase activity towards bilirubin and the effect of premature birth on this activity in the human liver. Biochem J 1981;196(1):257–60.

21. Gartner LM. On the question of the relationship between breastfeeding and jaundice in the first 5 days of life. Semin Perinatol 1994;18(6):502–9.

22. Gourley GR. Breast-feeding, neonatal jaundice and kernicterus. Semin Neonatol 2002;7(2):135–41.

23. Boyer DB, Vidyasagar D. Serum indirect bilirubin levels and meconium passage in early fed normal newborns. Nurse Res 1987;36(3):174–8.

24. Maisels MJ. What's in a name? Physiologic and pathologic jaundice: the conundrum of defining normal bilirubin levels in the newborn. Pediatrics 2006;118(2):805–7.

25. Hardy RC, Drage JS, Jackson EC. The first year of life: the collaborative perinatal project of the National Institutes of Neurological and Communicative Disorders and Stroke. Baltimore (MD): John Hopkins University Press; 1979.

26. Maisels MJ, Kring E. Transcutaneous bilirubin levels in the first 96 hours in a normal newborn population of > or = 35 weeks' gestation. Pediatrics 2006;117(4):1169–73.

27. Bhutani VK, Johnson L, Sivieri EM. Predictive ability of a predischarge hour-specific serum bilirubin for subsequent significant hyperbilirubinemia in healthy term and near-term newborns. Pediatrics 1999;103(1):6–14.

28. Newman TB, Escobar GJ, Gonzales VM, et al. Frequency of neonatal bilirubin testing and hyperbilirubinemia in a large health maintenance organization. Pediatrics 1999;104(5 Pt 2):1198–203.

29. Maisels MJ, Fanaroff AA, Stevenson DK, et al. Serum bilirubin levels in an international, multiracial newborn population. Pediatr Res 1999;45(4 Pt 2):167A.

30. Juretschke LJ. Kernicterus: still a concern. Neonatal Netw 2005;24(2):7–19.

31. Maisels MJ. Neonatal hyperbilirubinemia. In: Klaus MH, Fanaroff AA, editors. Care of the high-risk neonate. 5th edition. Philadelphia: WB Saunders Company; 2001. p. 324–62.

32. Saigal S, Lunyk O, Bennett KJ, et al. Serum bilirubin levels in breast- and formula-fed infants in the first 5 days of life. Can Med Assoc J 1982;127(10):985–9.

33. Okolo AA, Omene JA, Scott-Emuakpor AB. Physiologic jaundice in the Nigerian neonate. Biol Neonate 1988;53(3):132–7.

34. Maisels MJ, Kring E. Transcutaneous bilirubinometry decreases the need for serum bilirubin measurements and saves money. Pediatrics 1997;99(4):599–601.

35. de Almeida MF, Draque CM. Neonatal jaundice and breastfeeding. NeoReviews 2007;8(7):e282–8. Available at: http://neoreviews.aappublications.org/cgi/content/full/neoreviews;8/7/e282. Accessed June 27, 2008.

36. Maisels MJ. Neonatal jaundice. Pediatr Rev 2006;27(12):443–54.

37. Maisels MJ, Gifford K. Normal serum bilirubin levels in the newborn and the effect of breastfeeding. Pediatrics 1986;78(5):837–43.

38. Schneider AP. Breast milk jaundice in the newborn: a real entity. JAMA 1986;255(23):3270–4.

39. Jaundice. Centers for Disease Control and Prevention Web site. Available at: http://www.cdc.gov/breastfeeding/disease/jaundice.htm. Accessed June 21, 2008.

40. Fevery J. Fasting hyperbilirubinemia: unraveling the mechanism involved. Gastroenterology 1997;113(5):1798–800.

41. Gartner U, Goeser T, Wolkoff AW. Effect of fasting on the uptake of bilirubin and sulfobromophthalein by the isolated perfused rat liver. Gastroenterology 1997;113(5):1707–13.

42. De Carvalho M, Robertson S, Klaus M. Fecal bilirubin excretion and serum bilirubin concentrations in breast-fed and bottle-fed infants. J Pediatr 1985;107(5):786–90.

43. Yamauchi Y, Yamanouchi I. Breast-feeding frequency during the first 24 hours after birth in full-term neonates. Pediatrics 1990;86(2):171–5.

44. De Carvalho M, Klaus MH, Merkatz RB. Frequency of breastfeeding and serum bilirubin concentration. Am J Dis Child 1982;136(8):737–8.

45. Yoshioka H, Iseki K, Fujita K. Development and differences of intestinal flora in the neonatal period in breast-fed and bottle-fed infants. Pediatrics 1983;72(3):317–21.

46. Frank CG, Frank PH. Jaundice. In: Merenstein GB, Gardner LS, editors. Handbook of neonatal intensive care. 6th edition. St. Louis (MO): Mosby Elsevier; 2006. p. 548–68.

47. Kernicterus in full-term infants: United States, 1994–1998. MMWR Morb Mortal Wkly Rep 2001;50(23):491–4.

48. Kaplan M, Hammerman C. Glucose-6-phosphate dehydrogenase deficiency: a worldwide potential cause of severe neonatal hyperbilirubinemia.

NeoReviews 2000;1:e32–9. Available at: http://neoreviews.aappublications.org/cgi/content/full/neoreviews;1/2/e32. Accessed June 27, 2008.

49. Kaplan M, Hammerman C. Glucose-6-phosphate dehydrogenase deficiency: a hidden risk for kernicterus. Semin Perinatol 2004;28(5):356–64.

50. WHO Working Group. Glucose-6-phosphate dehydrogenase deficiency. Bull World Health Organ 1989;67:610–1.

51. Johnson LH, Bhutani VK, Brown AK. System-based approach to management of neonatal jaundice and prevention of kernicterus. J Pediatr 2002;140(4):396–403.

52. Cashore WJ. Bilirubin metabolism and toxicity in the newborn. In: Polin RA, Fox WW, Abman SH, editors. Fetal and neonatal physiology. 3rd edition. Philadelphia: Saunders; 2004. p. 1199–210.

53. Fox IJ, Chowdhury JR, Kaufman SS, et al. Treatment of the Crigler-Najjar syndrome type I with hepatocyte transplantation. N Engl J Med 1998;338(20):1422–6.

54. Chowdhury JR, Chowdhury NR, Strom SC, et al. Human hepatocyte transplantation: gene therapy and more? Pediatrics 1998;102(3 Pt 1):647–8.

55. Rubaltelli FF, Guerrini P, Reddi E, et al. Tin-protoporphyrin in the management of children with Crigler-Najjar disease. Pediatrics 1989;84(4):728–31.

56. Kappas A. A method for interdicting the development of severe jaundice in newborns by inhibiting the production of bilirubin. Pediatrics 2004;113(1 Pt 1):119–23.

57. Van der Veere CN, Jansen PL, Sinaasappel M, et al. Oral calcium phosphate: a new therapy for Crigler-Najjar disease? Gastroenterology 1997;112(2):455–62.

58. Bancroft JD, Kreamer B, Gourley GR. Gilbert syndrome accelerates development of neonatal jaundice. J Pediatr 1998;132(4):656–60.

59. Laforgia N, Faienza MF, Rinaldi A, et al. Neonatal hyperbilirubinemia and Gilbert's syndrome. J Perinat Med 2002;30(2):166–9.

60. Venigalla S, Gourley GR. Neonatal cholestasis. Semin Perinatol 2004;28(5):348–55.

61. McLin VA, Balistreri WF. Approach to neonatal cholestasis. In: Walker WA, Goulet O, Kleinman RE, et al, editors. Pediatric gastrointestinal disease: pathophysiology, diagnosis, management. 4th edition. Hamilton (Ontario, Canada): BC Decker, Inc.; 2004. p. 1079–93.

62. McKiernan PJ. Neonatal cholestasis. Semin Neonatol 2002;7(2):153–65.

63. Schmorl G. Zur kenntnis des ikterus neonatorum, insbesondere der dabei auftretenden gehirnveranderungen [German]. Verh Dtsch Ges Pathol 1904;6:109–15.

64. Johnson L, Brown AK, Bhutani VK. Bind: a clinical score for bilirubin induced neurologic dysfunction in newborns. Pediatrics 1999;104:746–7.

65. Ip S, Chung M, Kulig J, et al. An evidence-based review of important issues concerning neonatal hyperbilirubinemia. Pediatrics 2004;114(1):e130–53.

66. Andersen DH, Blanc WA, Crozier DN. A difference in mortality rate and incidence of kernicterus among premature infants allotted to two prophylactic antibacterial regimens. Pediatrics 1956;18(4):614–25.

67. Odell GB. Studies in kernicterus. I. The protein binding of bilirubin. J Clin Invest 1959;38(5):823–33.

68. Jardine DS, Rogers K. Relationship of benzyl alcohol to kernicterus, intraventricular hemorrhage, and mortality in preterm infants. Pediatrics 1989;83(2):153–60.

69. Volpe JJ. Bilirubin and brain injury. In: Neurology of the newborn. 4th edition. Philadelphia: WB Saunders Company; 2000. p. 521–64.

70. Dennery PA, Seidman DS, Stevenson DK. Neonatal hyperbilirubinemia. N Engl J Med 2001;344(8):581–90.

71. Newman TB, Liljestrand P, Jeremy RJ, et al. Outcomes among newborns with total serum bilirubin levels of 25 mg per deciliter or more. N Engl J Med 2006;354(18):1889–900.

72. Penn AA, Enzmann DR, Hahn JS, et al. Kernicterus in a full term infant. Pediatrics 1994;93(6 Pt 1):1003–6.

73. Maisels MJ, Newman TB. Kernicterus in otherwise healthy, breast-fed term newborns. Pediatrics 1995;96(4 Pt 1):730–3.

74. Ebbesen F. Recurrence of kernicterus in term and near-term infants in Denmark. Acta Paediatr 2000;89(10):1213–7.

75. Govaert P, Lequin M, Swarte R, et al. Changes in globus pallidus with (pre)term kernicterus. Pediatrics 2003;112(6 Pt 1):1256–63.

76. Slusher TM, Vreman HJ, McLaren DW, et al. Glucose-6-phosphate dehydrogenase deficiency and carboxyhemoglobin concentrations associated with bilirubin-related morbidity and death in Nigerian infants. J Pediatr 1995;126(1):102–8.

77. Murki S, Kumar P, Majumdar S, et al. Risk factors for kernicterus in term babies with non-hemolytic jaundice. Indian Pediatr 2001;38(7):757–62.

78. Nair PAK, Al Khussiby SM. Kernicterus and G6PD deficiency: a case series from Oman. J Trop Pediatr 2003;49:74–7.

79. Stanley TV. A case of kernicterus in New Zealand: a predictable tragedy? J Paediatr Child Health 1997;33:451–3.

80. Watchko JF. Vigintiphobia revisited. Pediatrics 2005;115(6):1747–53.

81. Eaton AP. Early postpartum discharge: recommendations from a preliminary report to Congress. Pediatrics 2001;107(2):400–3.

82. Li R, Zhao Z, Mokdad A, et al. Prevalence of breastfeeding in the United States: the 2001 national immunization survey. Pediatrics 2003;111(5 Part 2):1198–201.

83. American Academy of Pediatrics Subcommittee on Hyperbilirubinemia. Neonatal jaundice and kernicterus. Pediatrics 2001;108(3):763–5.

84. Gartner LM, Snyder RN, Chabon RS, et al. Kernicterus: high incidence in premature infants with low serum bilirubin concentrations. Pediatrics 1970;45(6):906–17.

85. Watchko JF, Oski FA. Kernicterus in preterm newborns: past, present, and future. Pediatrics 1992;90(5):707–15.

86. Watchko JF, Maisels MJ. Jaundice in low birthweight infants: pathobiology and outcome. Arch Dis Child Fetal Neonatal Ed 2003;88(6):F455–8.

87. Maisels MJ, Watchko JF. Treatment of jaundice in low birthweight infants. Arch Dis Child Fetal Neonatal Ed 2003;88(6):F459–63.

88. National Institute of Child Health and Human Development. Randomized, controlled trial of phototherapy for neonatal hyperbilirubinemia: executive summary. Pediatrics 1985;75(2 Pt 2):385–6.

89. Kramer LI. Advancement of dermal icterus in the jaundiced newborn. Am J Dis Child 1969;118(3):454–8.

90. Johnson L, Bhutani VK. Guidelines for management of the jaundiced term and near-term infant. Clin Perinatol 1998;25(3):555–74, viii.

91. Moyer VA, Ahn C, Sneed S. Accuracy of clinical judgment in neonatal jaundice. Arch Pediatr Adolesc Med 2000;154(4):391–4.

92. Sykes E, Epstein E. Laboratory measurement of bilirubin. Clin Perinatol 1990;17(2):397–416.

93. Doumas BT, Wu TW. The measurement of bilirubin fractions in serum. Crit Rev Clin Lab Sci 1991; 28(5-6):415–45.

94. Vreman HJ, Verter J, Oh W, et al. Interlaboratory variability of bilirubin measurements. Clin Chem 1996;42(6 Pt 1):869–73.

95. Doumas BT, Eckfeldt JH. Errors in measurement of total bilirubin: a perennial problem. Clin Chem 1996;42(6 Pt 1):845–8.

96. Lo SF, Doumas BT, Ashwood ER. Performance of bilirubin determinations in US laboratories: revisited. Clin Chem 2004;50(1):190–4.

97. Gourley GR. Bilirubin metabolism and kernicterus. Adv Pediatr 1997;44:173–229.

98. Eidelman AI, Schimmel MS, Algur N, et al. Capillary and venous bilirubin values: they are different–and how!. Am J Dis Child 1989;143(6):642.

99. Leslie GI, Philips JB III, Cassady G. Capillary and venous bilirubin values: are they really different? Am J Dis Child 1987;141(11):1199–200.

100. Ahlfors CE. Criteria for exchange transfusion in jaundiced newborns. Pediatrics 1994;93(3):488–94.

101. Ahlfors CE, Wennberg RP. Bilirubin-albumin binding and neonatal jaundice. Semin Perinatol 2004;28:334–9.

102. Wennberg RP, Ahlfors CE, Bhutani VK, et al. Toward understanding kernicterus: a challenge to improve the management of jaundiced newborns. Pediatrics 2006;117(2):474–85.

103. Amin SB. Clinical assessment of bilirubin-induced neurotoxicity in premature infants. Semin Perinatol 2004;28(5):340–7.

104. McDonagh AF, Maisels MJ. Bilirubin unbound: deja vu all over again? Pediatrics 2006;117(2):523–5.

105. Hanko E. Unbound bilirubin and risk assessment in the jaundiced newborn: possibilities and limitations. Pediatrics 2006;117(2):526–7.

106. Blackmon LR, Fanaroff AA, Raju TN. Research on prevention of bilirubin-induced brain injury and kernicterus: National Institute of Child Health and Human Development conference executive summary, 2003. Pediatrics 2004;114(1):229–33.

107. Grohmann K, Roser M, Rolinski B, et al. Bilirubin measurement for neonates: comparison of 9 frequently used methods. Pediatrics 2006;117(4):1174–83.

108. Bhutani VK, Gourley GR, Adler S, et al. Noninvasive measurement of total serum bilirubin in a multiracial predischarge newborn population to assess the risk of severe hyperbilirubinemia. Pediatrics 2000;106(2): E17. Available at: http://pediatrics.aappublications. org/cgi/reprint/106/2/e17. Accessed June 12, 2008.

109. Briscoe L, Clark S, Yoxall CW. Can transcutaneous bilirubinometry reduce the need for blood tests in jaundiced full term babies? Arch Dis Child Fetal Neonatal Ed 2002;86(3):F190–2.

110. Ebbesen F, Rasmussen LM, Wimberley PD. A new transcutaneous bilirubinometer, bilicheck, used in the neonatal intensive care unit and the maternity ward. Acta Paediatr 2002;91(2):203–11.

111. Rubaltelli FF, Gourley GR, Loskamp N, et al. Transcutaneous bilirubin measurement: a multicenter evaluation of a new device. Pediatrics 2001;107(6):1264–71.

112. Yasuda S, Itoh S, Isobe K, et al. New transcutaneous jaundice device with two optical paths. J Perinat Med 2003;31(1):81–8.

113. Maisels MJ, Ostrea EM Jr, Touch S, et al. Evaluation of a new transcutaneous bilirubinometer. Pediatrics 2004;113(6):1628–35.

114. Slusher TM, Angyo IA, Bode-Thomas F, et al. Transcutaneous bilirubin measurements and serum total bilirubin levels in indigenous African infants. Pediatrics 2004;113(6):1636–41.

115. Engle WD, Jackson GL, Sendelbach D, et al. Assessment of a transcutaneous device in the evaluation of neonatal hyperbilirubinemia in a primarily Hispanic population. Pediatrics 2002;110(1 Pt 1): 61–7.

116. Jaundice meter JM-103 [product catalogue]. Konica Minolta Web site. Available at: http://www. konicaminolta.com/instruments/download/catalog/ medical/pdf/jm103_e7.pdf. Accessed July 2, 2008.

117. Stevenson DK, Fanaroff AA, Maisels MJ, et al. Prediction of hyperbilirubinemia in near-term and term infants. Pediatrics 2001;108(1):31–9.

118. Newman TB, Xiong B, Gonzales VM, et al. Prediction and prevention of extreme neonatal hyperbilirubinemia

in a mature health maintenance organization. Arch Pediatr Adolesc Med 2000;154(11):1140–7.

119. Maisels MJ, Kring E. Length of stay, jaundice, and hospital readmission. Pediatrics 1998;101(6):995–8.

120. Keren R, Luan X, Friedman S, et al. A comparison of alternative risk-assessment strategies for predicting significant neonatal hyperbilirubinemia in term and near-term infants. Pediatrics 2008;121(1):e170–9.

121. Cremer RJ, Perryman PW, Richards DH. Influence of light on the hyperbilirubinaemia of infants. Lancet 1958;1(7030):1094–7.

122. Maisels MJ, Kring EA, DeRidder J. Randomized controlled trial of light-emitting diode phototherapy. J Perinatol 2007;27(9):565–7.

123. Tan KL. The pattern of bilirubin response to phototherapy for neonatal hyperbilirubinaemia. Pediatr Res 1982;16(8):670–4.

124. Tan KL. Phototherapy for neonatal jaundice. Clin Perinatol 1991;18(3):423–39.

125. Holtrop PC, Ruedisueli K, Maisels MJ. Double versus single phototherapy in low birth weight newborns. Pediatrics 1992;90(5):674–7.

126. Tan KL. Comparison of the efficacy of fiberoptic and conventional phototherapy for neonatal hyperbilirubinemia. J Pediatr 1994;125(4):607–12.

127. Maisels MJ. A primer on phototherapy for the jaundiced newborn. Contemp Pediatr 2005;22(6). passim. 38,40,44,47,48,53,54,57.

128. Stokowski LA. Fundamentals of phototherapy for neonatal jaundice. Adv Neonatal Care 2006;6(6): 303–12.

129. Mills JF, Tudehope D. Fibreoptic phototherapy for neonatal jaundice. NICHD Cochrane neonatal Web site. Available at: http://www.nichd.nih.gov/cochrane/Mills/Review.htm. Accessed July 2, 2008.

130. Tonz O, Vogt J, Filippini L, et al [Severe light dermatosis following photo therapy in a newborn infant with congenital erythropoietic urophyria]. Helv Paediatr Acta 1975;30(1):47–56, German.

131. Kearns GL, Williams BJ, Timmons OD. Fluorescein phototoxicity in a premature infant. J Pediatr 1985; 107(5):796–8.

132. Pezzati M, Fusi F, Dani C, et al. Changes in skin temperature of hyperbilirubinemic newborns under phototherapy: conventional versus fiberoptic device. Am J Perinatol 2002;19(8):439–44.

133. Dollberg S, Atherton HD, Hoath SB. Effect of different phototherapy lights on incubator characteristics and dynamics under three modes of servocontrol. Am J Perinatol 1995;12(1):55–60.

134. Grunhagen DJ, de Boer MG, de Beaufort AJ, et al. Transepidermal water loss during halogen spotlight phototherapy in preterm infants. Pediatr Res 2002; 51(3):402–5.

135. Maayan-Metzger A, Yosipovitch G, Hadad E, et al. Transepidermal water loss and skin hydration in preterm infants during phototherapy. Am J Perinatol 2001;18(7):393–6.

136. Csoma Z, Kemeny L, Olah J. Phototherapy for neonatal jaundice. N Engl J Med 2008;358(23):2523–4.

137. Csoma Z, Hencz P, Orvos H, et al. Neonatal blue-light phototherapy could increase the risk of dysplastic nevus development. Pediatrics 2007; 119(6):1036–7.

138. Garg AK, Prasad RS, Hifzi IA. A controlled trial of high-intensity double-surface phototherapy on a fluid bed versus conventional phototherapy in neonatal jaundice. Pediatrics 1995;95(6):914–6.

139. Hansen TW. Acute management of extreme neonatal jaundice: the potential benefits of intensified phototherapy and interruption of enterohepatic bilirubin circulation. Acta Paediatr 1997;86(8):843–6.

140. Maisels MJ, Kring E. Rebound in serum bilirubin level following intensive phototherapy. Arch Pediatr Adolesc Med 2002;156(7):669–72.

141. Kaplan M, Kaplan E, Hammerman C, et al. Post-phototherapy neonatal bilirubin rebound: a potential cause of significant hyperbilirubinaemia. Arch Dis Child 2006;91(1):31–4.

142. Steiner LA, Bizzarro MJ, Ehrenkranz RA, et al. A decline in the frequency of neonatal exchange transfusions and its effect on exchange-related morbidity and mortality. Pediatrics 2007;120(1):27–32.

143. Maisels MJ. Phototherapy: traditional and nontraditional. J Perinatol 2001;21(Suppl 1):S93–7.

144. Rubo J, Albrecht K, Lasch P, et al. High-dose intravenous immune globulin therapy for hyperbilirubinemia caused by Rh hemolytic disease. J Pediatr 1992;121(1):93–7.

145. Dagoglu T, Ovali F, Samanci N, et al. High dose intravenous immunoglobulin therapy for haemolytic disease. J Int Med Res 1995;23(4):264–71.

146. Voto LS, Sexer H, Ferreiro G, et al. Neonatal administration of high-dose intravenous immunoglobulin in rhesus hemolytic disease. J Perinat Med 1995; 23(6):443–51.

147. Hammermann C, Kaplan M. Recent developments in the management of neonatal hyperbilirubinemia. NeoReviews 2000;1(2):e19–24. Available at: http://neoreviews.aappublications.org/cgi/content/full/neoreviews;1/2/e19. Accessed June 27, 2008.

148. Gottstein R, Cooke RW. Systematic review of intravenous immunoglobulin in haemolytic disease of the newborn. Arch Dis Child Fetal Neonatal Ed 2003;88(1):F6–10.

149. Valaes T, Petmezaki S, Henschke C, et al. Control of jaundice in preterm newborns by an inhibitor of bilirubin production: studies with tin-mesoporphyrin. Pediatrics 1994;93(1):1–11.

150. Martinez JC, Garcia HO, Otheguy LE, et al. Control of severe hyperbilirubinemia in full-term newborns with the inhibitor of bilirubin production Sn-mesoporphyrin. Pediatrics 1999;103(1):1–5.

Sepsis in the Neonate

Sandra L. Gardner, RN, MS, CNS, PNP

KEYWORDS

- Sepsis • Neonate • Septicemia • Neonatal infections
- Transplacental/intrapartum infections
- Congenital viral infections

In the neonatal intensive care unit (ICU), critical care nurses who are not advanced practice nurses cannot make the medical diagnosis of infection/sepsis in the neonate. Even so, the critical care nurse has an important role in dealing with sepsis/infection. The nurse must (1) have a high index of suspicion about the risk of infection, (2) be able to recognize septic/infected newborns, (3) report related concerns to the physician or advanced practice nurse, and (4) be prepared to advocate on behalf of the infant to ensure timely diagnostic workup and empiric antibiotics.

DEFINITIONS

Septicemia, commonly called blood poisoning, is a generalized bacterial infection in the bloodstream. Neonatal infections, which may be caused by bacteria, viruses, or fungi, occur as early or late infections and their timing gives care providers clues for determining causative agents. Transplacental/intrapartum infections occur in utero and manifest within the first 3 days ($\leq$72 hours) of life. These early-onset infections are associated with high morbidity and mortality.[1] Late-onset infections may occur as early as 3 days of age, but more commonly occur after the first week of life. For late-preterm and term infants discharged within the first 48 to 72 hours of life, parents, rather than the neonatal nurse, take on the responsibility of recognizing when their infant is "sick" and needs to be examined by a health care provider.

INCIDENCE

The World Health Organization (WHO) estimates that each year 4 million newborns worldwide die during the neonatal period.[2] Seventy-five percent of these deaths occur during the first week of life, and 25% to 45% of neonatal deaths occur the first day of life.[3,4] Neonatal deaths are mainly caused by severe infections (36%), prematurity (28%) and birth defects (7%).[2] In the United States, 1 to 5 of every 1000 live births result in neonatal infection. Neonates with certain risk factors are at higher risk for developing infection/sepsis (**Fig. 1**). Causative agents in neonatal sepsis are listed in **Fig. 2**. The Centers for Disease Control and Prevention estimates that, for every 141 babies born in the United States each year, 1 dies of infection in the first year of life. That comes to 30,000 newborn deaths, including 20,000 in the first month of life. Before the use of antibiotics, mortality rates for newborns with infection/sepsis were 95% to 100%; after use of antibiotics, mortality rates range from 13% to 45%.[1] Lower mortality rates are the result of earlier case-finding, timely diagnostic evaluation, and initiation of empiric antibiotic therapy. Both inpatient and outpatient neonatal care requires timely diagnosis and therapy; delay is associated with worsening morbidity and mortality.[5]

PREVENTION

Neonatal nurses are the first line of defense in preventing infections, in recognizing subtle signs and symptoms, and in advocating that the newborn receive a timely diagnostic workup and empiric antibiotic therapy.[5] Knowledgeable nurses are able to recognize an individual infant's risk factors for infection and approach assessment and interaction with newborns with a high level of suspicion regarding infection. The primary nurse teaches parents how to interact with their newborn, interpret cues, and recognize deviations from normal neonatal behavior.

Hand hygiene (hand rubs/hand washing) and universal precautions are the cornerstone of infection prevention and control. Using accepted infection control principles, practices, control

E-mail address: gardnerslconsult@aol.com

Crit Care Nurs Clin N Am 21 (2009) 121–141
doi:10.1016/j.ccell.2008.11.002
0899-5885/08/$ – see front matter © 2009 Elsevier Inc. All rights reserved.

Immature immune system in preterm/ term newborns—less nonspecific (inflammatory) immunity, specific (humoral) immunity and no local inflammatory reaction to portal of entry of infection

Signs and symptoms vague and nonspecific—mimic signs and symptoms of other common morbidities

Sex difference---male infants 2:1 higher occurrence than females

Method of feeding---breast feeding protective

Prematurity---less/ no passive immunity which is gestational age specific; 3-5 fold increased risk

Multiple pathways of acquiring infection—transplacental, perinatal and postpartal Antibiotic use

Low birth weight (LBW);intrauterine growth restricted (IUGR)—underweight/ malnourished newborns, of any gestation

Maternal infection---history of maternal infection increases newborn's risk of also being infected

Intrapartum complications---premature rupture of membranes, preterm onset of labor, maternal temperature; internal monitor electrode; resuscitation

Congenital malformations---birth defects such as gastroschisis, myelomenigocele

Procedures---any invasive procedure (i.e. PIV; UAC/UVC; PICC; ETT; LP; surgery)

Fig. 1. Risk factors associated with an increased risk for neonatal infection/sepsis. *Data from* Gardner SL. "How will I know if my newborn is sick?" Nurse Currents 2008;2(2):1–5.

measures, and techniques in the hospital prevents and controls the spread of infectious disease.[1] Hand hygiene programs increase compliance and are associated with decreased risk for nosocomial infections in very low birth weight infants.[6]

Early-Onset Sepsis
Common Organisms:
  Group B Streptococcus (GBS)
  Escherichia coli
  Haemophilus influenzae (type b/nontypeable)
  Coagulase-negative *Staphylococcus* (CONS)
Unusual Organisms:
  Staphylococcus aureus
  Neisseria meningitides
  Streptococcus pneumoniae
  Listeria monocytogenes
Rare Organisms:
  Klebsiella pneumoniae
  Pseudomonas aeruginosa
  Enterobacter species
  Serratia marcescens
  Anaerobic species *(Bacteriodes;Clostridium)*
  Salmonella
  Citrobacter
  Proteus

Late-Onset Sepsis
  Coagulase-negative *Staphylococcus* (CONS)
  Escherichia coli
  Klebsiella species
  Enterobacter species
  Candida species
  Malassezia furfur
  Other enteric organisms
  Group B Streptococcus (GBS)
  Staphylococcus aureus
  Methicillin-resistant *Staphylococcus aureus* (MRSA)
  Staphylococcus epidermidis

Fig. 2. Causative agents in neonatal sepsis. *Data from* Venkatesh M, Merenstein GB, Adams K, et al. Infection in the neonate. In: Merenstein GB, Gardner SL, editors. Handbook of neonatal Intensive Care, 6th edition, St. Louis (MO): Mosby; 2006. p. 569–93; American Academy of Pediatrics. Influenza. In: Red book: 2006 Report of the Committee on Infectious Diseases, 27th edition, Elk Grove, IL, AAP; Newton O, English M. Young infant sepsis: aetiology, antibiotic susceptibility and clinical signs. Royal Society of Tropical Medicine and Hygiene 2007;101:959–66.

Whether in the newborn nursery or in the neonatal ICU, nurses are responsible for teaching new parents the importance of hand hygiene both in the hospital and after discharge. As advocates for their infant, parents must also be taught how to screen and restrict visitors who are "sick" with infectious diseases and be told of the importance of not taking neonates into crowds (eg, malls, church nurseries, childcare, children's parties). These strategies, along with breast-feeding, help protect infants and prevent infections after hospital discharge.[5]

SIGNS AND SYMPTOMS

Signs and symptoms of infection in the neonate are subtle, nonspecific, and mimic signs and symptoms of other neonatal morbidities (eg, hypoglycemia, hypothermia, respiratory distress, primary apnea of prematurity, neurologic conditions, cardiac disease) (**Fig. 3**). The key to better survival with less morbidity is early case-finding; this is one of the best reasons to have primary nursing. Most often, the neonate's primary nurse and the mother are the first to notice subtle changes in feeding behavior, alertness, and muscle tone. Even if all the "numbers" (ie, vital signs) are within normal range, there is often a feeling by mother, the primary nurse, or both that "something is wrong" or "the baby isn't doing well." When dealing with a newborn, it is always wise to err on the side of caution and heed these subtle signs and vague complaints; otherwise, by the time the symptoms become "obvious," a baby can be moribund and overwhelmingly septic.[7]

The primary nurse who consistently cares for an infant and plans and directs care with the parents has a high index of suspicion when the infant presents with subtle and vague symptoms. As a patient advocate, the primary nurse notifies the physician

Temperature instability: Hypothermia or Hyperthermia
Respiratory distress: Tachypnea, apnea, cyanosis, grunting/ flaring/ retracting
Cardiovascular changes: Tachycardia, bradycardia, hypotension, pallor, poor
                        peripheral perfusion, prolonged capillary refill time, weak
                        pulses, decreased urine output
Lethargy/ irritability/ seizures
Feeding abnormalities: Poor feeding, vomiting, increase in residuals, abdominal
                       distention, diarrhea
Jaundice: Increase in direct and /or indirect bilirubin
Skin changes: Purpura, rash, erythema, petechiae
Metabolic changes: Acidosis (metabolic and /or respiratory), hypoglycemia,
                   hypoxia

Fig. 3. Signs and symptoms of neonatal sepsis. *Data from* Venkatesh M, Merenstein GB, Adams K, et al. Infection in the neonate. In: Merenstein GB, Gardner SL, editors. Handbook of neonatal intensive care, 6th edition, St. Louis (MO), Mosby 2006. p. 569–93; Gardner SL. Late-preterm ("near-term") newborns: a neonatal nursing challenge. Nurse Currents 2007;1(1):1–7. Gardner SL, Brown VD. "Near-term" deliveries and "near-term" infants: when almost isn't quite good enough!!©NPDPA, 2007. Nurse's Professional Development and Practice Association, LLC™. Available at: www.npdpa.com.

or advanced practice nurse of any signs or symptoms that could be related to infection. The nurse then advocates for prompt screening, immediate diagnostic workup, and timely therapy.

However, recognizing symptoms, reporting suspicions, and convincing others that a neonate may have an infection has always been a nursing challenge. Recently, for her doctoral dissertation, Lori Baas Rubarth[8] developed an objective, reliable, and valid scoring tool (**Fig. 4**) for neonatal sepsis/infection. Even though her initial goal was to assist new nurses, her Scale of Sepsis (SOS) is relevant for all nurses using both clinical and laboratory data to assess a newborn for sepsis. Just as the Apgar score and the numerous pain tools used to assess the newborn give objective data, the SOS can be used as an objective tool to convince physicians (ie, pediatricians, family practice physicians, and neonatologists) and advanced practice nurses (ie, clinical specialists, family/neonatal/pediatric practitioners) that an individual infant should be evaluated for sepsis. Both inpatient and outpatient nurses can, in addition to collecting the perinatal/neonatal/pediatric history, use the eight clinical indicators in the SOS scale as part of their initial assessment of the newborn.

Although Rubarth initially intended to develop a diagnostic tool for neonatal sepsis, the SOS scale is an assessment, rather than a diagnostic, tool. In the testing phase, the SOS was shown to be a very nonspecific tool for diagnosing sepsis because the predictive validity of the tool was unacceptable.[5,8] For example, newborns with respiratory distress (ie, tachypnea, grunting, flaring and retracting) had a high SOS score, even though they did not have sepsis. The SOS is better at determining the absence, rather than the presence, of sepsis.

When using the SOS scale, the number of points for the laboratory markers and the number for clinical indicators are totaled for an individual newborn. The maximum possible score is 55 with 35 points for clinical indicators and 20 points for laboratory markers.[8] A total clinical score less than 10 indicates that the newborn does not have sepsis—a negative predictive value of 97%.[8,9] Any neonate with a total clinical score greater than 10 is considered "sick," possibly with sepsis. A clinical score greater than 10 is also an indicator of the need for further diagnostic evaluation (ie, complete blood cell count, differential and platelets; arterial blood gas; C-reactive protein [CRP]). Even though the SOS scale does not clearly indicate infection, it assists nurses in recognizing the clinical pattern of sepsis and in interpreting complete blood cell count results. The SOS has been crafted into a clinical practice tool with documentation forms (available at: www.npdpa.com).

If recognizing signs and symptoms of infection in a newborn is difficult for professional caregivers, it is even more difficult for parents who are unfamiliar with normal newborn behavior and subtle signs of neonatal distress. Before discharge, every parent must be taught how to recognize a "sick" newborn, must be given written instructions of what a sick newborn looks like and how it behaves, and be provided clear instructions on whom to notify if the newborn shows signs of sickness. This is especially critical for any neonate with risk factors (see **Fig. 1**). The WHO states that improving identification of infants who are severely ill (and in danger of dying) within the first week of life is of major public health importance worldwide.[3] To clarify signs and symptoms of neonatal sepsis, the WHO conducted a large multisite study of the clinical features and causes of serious bacterial disease from 1990 to 1992 in infants less than 2 months old. The WHO developed an algorithm—Integrated Management of Childhood Illness (IMCI)—based on the study.[10–17] This initial

Newborn Scale Of Sepsis (SOS)
Rubarth ©2005

Name_____ Date of Exam_____ Age at Exam_____(hours)

Laboratory Findings:	**Score**
White Blood Cell Count	
(<5,000 = **5** , > 30,000 = **2**, 5,000-30,000 = **0**)	☐
Immature:Total Neutrophil Ratio	
(> 0.3 = **5**, 0.2-0.3 = **3**, < 0.2 = **0**)	☐
Platelet Count	
(<100,000 = **3**, ≥ 100,000 = **0**)	☐
Blood Acidity	
(pH < 7.25 = **2**, pH 7.25-7.34 = **1**, pH normal 7.35-7.45 = **0**)	☐
Absolute Neutrophil Count	
(<1000 = **5**, 1000-2000 = **3**, > 2000 = **0**)	☐

Clinical Indicators:	
Skin Color	
(Ashen/Grey = **5**, Dusky = **3**, Mottled = **2**, Acrocyanosis = **1**, Pink = **0**)	☐
Perfusion (Cap. Refill)	
(Poor> 7 sec = **5**, Moderate 6-7 sec = **3**, Fair 4-5 sec = **1**, Good < 4 sec = **0**)	☐
Muscle Tone	
(Flaccid = **5**, Low tone = **3**, Good tone = **0**)	☐
Responsiveness to Pain	
(No response = **5**, Some response (withdrawal) = **2**, Active Crying = **0**)	☐
Respiratory Distress	
(Present with grunting = **5**, Present no grunting = **3**, None = **0**)	☐
Respiratory Rate	
(Respiratory rate ≥ 100 = **5**, RR 60-99 = **3**, RR < 60 = **0**)	☐
Temperature	
(Low temp < 97° F = **3**, High temp > 99° F = **2**, Normal 97-99° F. = **0**)	☐
Apnea	
(Present = **2**, Absent = **0**)	☐

Total Score _____

Fig. 4. Newborn Scale of Sepsis. A total clinical score less than 10 indicates that the newborn does not have sepsis—a negative predictive value of 97%. Any neonate with a total clinical score greater than 10 is considered "sick," possibly with sepsis. A clinical score greater than 10 is also an indicator of the need for further diagnostic evaluation. (*From* Rubarth LB. Nursing patterns of knowing in assessment of newborn sepsis [doctoral dissertation], University of Arizona, 2005; with permission.)

IMCI guideline did not cover ill newborns in the first week of life, the time when the majority of neonatal morbidity occurs. The WHO then conducted a more recent study to provide evidence to support an IMCI referral checklist for 0 to 7 days of life and to improve existing guidelines for 7 to 59 days of age.[3] From seven international study sites, the most common diagnoses (for 0–6-day olds) requiring hospitalization (excluding jaundice) were (1) severe infections (eg, sepsis, pneumonia, meningitis), (2) prematurity and low birth weight, and (3) birth asphyxia. Physiologic jaundice, low birth weight, and localized infections were the most common diagnoses not requiring hospitalization.

From an initial list of 20 signs/symptoms of newborn illness, 7 were found to be independent clinical predictors of severe illness requiring hospitalization for both 0- to 7-day-old neonates/infants and for 7- to 59-day-old neonates/infants (**Fig. 5**). In the WHO study, mothers or other caretakers had already decided that these infants were ill and needed to be seen by a health care provider. The WHO study resulted in the development of an algorithm intended for all infants less than 2 months of age brought to health facilities for an

History of feeding difficulty
Movement only when stimulated
Temperature < 35.5C
Temperature ≥ 37.5C
Respiratory rate > 60 breaths/ minute
Severe chest indrawing (retractions)
History of convulsions

Fig. 5. Signs and symptoms predictive of serious illness and the need for hospitalization in infants up to 59 days old. *Data from* The Young Infants Clinical Signs Study Group. Clinical signs that predict severe illness in children under age 2 months: a multi-center study. Lancet 2008;37:135.

illness. The presence of *any one sign* in **Fig. 5** has high sensitivity and specificity for severe illness requiring hospitalization in the first 2 months of life. To assist parents in early recognition of neonatal illness, evidence-based discharge teaching for parents should include instructions to watch for any of these highly reliable signs/symptoms. The Nurse's Professional Development & Practice Association has developed for discharge teaching of parents a written tool, "How Will I Know if My Baby is Sick?" This material includes a description of normal newborn behavior as well as a description of each of the signs/symptoms in **Fig. 5** (available at: www.npdpa.com).

DIAGNOSIS

Congenital viral infections are outlined in **Table 1**. Acquired bacterial, viral, and fungal infections are outlined in **Table 2**.

Diagnostic workup (**Fig. 6**) for sepsis is required in all neonates exhibiting signs/symptoms of sepsis and/or who are at increased risk for sepsis (see **Fig. 1**). However, because there is no laboratory test with 100% sensitivity and 100% specificity for neonatal sepsis, laboratory tests that are normal do not rule out sepsis.[18,19] Standard diagnostic tests in the adult are not necessarily diagnostic in the neonate; a normal complete blood cell count does not mean that the individual neonate is not septic. For instance, complete blood cell count (with differential) results may be difficult to interpret because of variations in normal values based on birth weight, gestational age, postconceptual age, physiologic stress, and or intrapartum complications (eg, low Apgar scores due to hypoxia and perinatal depression; pregnancy-induced hypertension). If surface cultures are obtained, colonization, not necessarily the presence of active systemic infection, is documented. In the neonate, blood culture, the gold standard for diagnosing and detecting bacteremia, has a positive predictive value of only 36%

to 38%.[20] Even in the presence of neonatal sepsis, blood cultures are not always positive. In this nonverbal, vulnerable population, a combination of clinical and laboratory evidence is required to diagnose and treat the individual neonate suspected of being septic.[21]

Elements of the complete blood cell count, such as the white blood cell count, differential, and platelet count, may be associated with bacterial sepsis. Leukopenia, a low white blood cell count (<5000/μL), and neutropenia, a low absolute neutrophil count (<1750/μL), are predictive of bacteremia in the neonate.[22] The presence of neutropenia and an abnormal immature neutrophil–to–total neutrophil (I/T) ratio is most predictive of infection.[23] An I/T ratio of 0.2 or more has 100% sensitivity, 50% specificity, and 100% negative predictive value.[8] In addition, a low platelet count (<100,000), thrombocytopenia, is also associated with neonatal sepsis. However, a single laboratory test and result must not be relied upon; laboratory tests in the newborn are most useful when serial testing is performed and initial results are compared with follow-up tests at 12 to 24 hours.[1]

Newer laboratory tests may not be readily available or be sensitive or specific enough on their own to influence clinical decisions about neonatal sepsis.[1,24–26] Acute-phase reactants are diagnostic markers for infection. CRP, an acute-phase reactant, is elevated in any acute inflammatory condition, including infection. However, studies on the efficacy of CRP are contradictory. Some show CRP to be a valuable screening tool for the diagnosis of neonatal sepsis[27–30] while other studies do not support the use of CRP because of low sensitivity and positive predictive values.[2,18,31–33] CRP is most valuable when serial testing and evaluation enables (1) "patterns" of increasing or decreasing levels to be evaluated, (2) the response to antibiotics to be monitored, and (3) the duration of treatment to be monitored.[33–35] Serum procalcitonin, an even newer test, is elevated in both early- and late-onset bacterial sepsis in the neonate, with a sensitivity of 92.6% and a specificity of 97.5% within the first 48 hours (in early-onset sepsis).[36]

The developmental immaturity of the immune system of the newborn prevents localization of infection. Therefore, meningitis is a frequent manifestation of sepsis in neonates, especially in very low birth weight preterms, in symptomatic infants, in early-onset group B streptococcus sepsis, and in late-onset sepsis.[1] However, meningitis may be present without overt signs of central nervous system infection.[24] Including lumbar puncture in sepsis workups is more common in neonatal care because meningitis is difficult to diagnose

Table 1
Congenital viral infections

Organism	Incidence	Perinatal Presentation	Neonatal Symptoms	Treatment	Parent Education
Toxoplasmosis	30% of newborns have congenital birth defects; 70%–90% are asymptomatic at birth	Asymptomatic in the mother	Intrauterine growth restricted; preterm; hydrocephalus; chorioretinitis; seizures; cerebral calcifications; hepatosplenomegaly; thrombocytopenia; jaundice; rash; general lympadenopathy	Congenitally infected neonates are treated with pyrimethamine (2 mg/kg/d) every 2–3 d and with sulfadiazine (100–200 mg/kg/d PO divided q 12 h) for a year; also supplemented daily with folic acid (1 mg/d); treatment for 1 y (instead of 1 mo) results in better neurologic, ocular, cognitive, and auditory outcomes[40]	Prevention: pregnant women to avoid contact with cat feces (changing litter box; gardening) and eating raw/ undercooked meat
Enteroviruses (eg, Coxsackie A and B), echovirus, poliomyelitis, and others	Frequent illness in infants and young children (hand-foot-mouth disease; conjunctivitis) spread by fecal-oral/ respiratory routes and from infected fomites; neonates who acquire infection (without maternal antibody) are at risk for severe disease with high mortality	Symptoms/disease processes include those related to respiratory functions (common cold, sore throat, stomatitis, pneumonia, herpangina, pleurodynia); the skin (exanthema); neurologic functions (aseptic meningitis, encephalitis, paralysis); gastrointestinal functions (vomiting, diarrhea, abdominal pain, hepatitis); ocular functions (acute hemorrhagic conjunctivitis); and cardiac functions	Signs and symptoms of neonatal sepsis	Immune globulin intravenous used in life-threatening neonatal infections	Pregnant women often are infected by young children, then infect their fetus; pregnant women and all childcare workers need to be taught the importance of universal/contact precautions and hand hygiene (hand washing/hand rubs), especially when changing diapers and dealing with respiratory, eye, and gastrointestinal secretions

Rubella	Decrease in incidence of 99% from prevaccine (measles mumps rubella [MMR] vaccine) era; <25 cases/y in United States	Maternal infection asymptomatic or only slight symptoms of "3-d measles"; first trimester infection is teratogenic to the fetus in 85% of cases	Intrauterine growth restricted; deafness; cataracts; jaundice; purpura (blueberry muffin syndrome); microcephaly; hepatosplenomegaly; bone lesions; chorio-retinitis; pneumonitis; cardiac defects (patent ductus arteriosis; pulmonic stenosis)	Prevention with measles, mumps, and rubella immunizations; supportive care	Discharge teaching: Infected infant/child sheds virus for 2–5 y in body fluids
Cytomegalovirus (CMV)	4%–5% of women carry virus; modes of transmission to neonate: (1) transplacental passage, (2) infected birth canal, (3) cytomegalovirus-positive breast-milk, (4) transfusion with cytomegalovirus-positive blood; 1% of all live-born infants are infected at birth and excrete cytomegalovirus	Majority of infected mothers are asymptomatic; neonatal sequelae of maternal cytomegalovirus infection most common with primary maternal infection	90% have no signs/symptoms at birth, but have later problems; 9% have transient thrombocytopenia (blueberry muffin syndrome); 1% are severely affected: intrauterine growth restricted; developmental delays; micro/hydrocephaly; seizures; jaundice; deafness; hepatosplenomegaly; chorioretinitis; cerebral calcifications	Antivirals: ganciclovir treatment of neonates with cytomegalovirus disease decreases progression of hearing impairment; ganciclovir not recommended for routine use because of insufficient efficacy data; oral ganciclovir is less effective than intravenous administration due to decreased bioavailability	Discharge teaching: Infected infant/child sheds virus for 2–5 y in body fluids; infection may occur from contact with the urine, saliva of preschool-age children[41]

(continued on next page)

Table 1
(continued)

Organism	Incidence	Perinatal Presentation	Neonatal Symptoms	Treatment	Parent Education
Herpes (herpes simplex virus [HSV])	1 of 3000–20,000 live births; increased incidence in preterm neonates; infected birth canal: 33%–50% risk of acquiring herpes (with maternal primary genital infection); <5% risk of acquiring herpes with maternal reactivated infection	Primary and recurrent infections may be asymptomatic or present with vaginal discharge, genital pain, shallow ulcers; 75% of neonates who contract herpes are born to mothers who have no history or clinical manifestations of herpes during pregnancy; 90% of pregnant women infected with herpes simplex virus are not aware of their infection	Initial symptoms appear at any time from birth to 4 wk of age; disseminated infection occurs earliest (in the first week of life); one third of neonatal herpes cases are localized, one third systemic, and one third central nervous system infections; localized skin lesions; systemic infections of the liver, lungs, central nervous system with disseminated herpes, which increases morbidity (severe neurologic sequelae)/mortality (25% with disseminated disease die despite therapy)	Antiviral: acyclovir (intravenous) 60 mg/kg/d in 3 divided doses for 14–21 d	Discharge teaching: good hand hygiene with antiseptic gels/hand washing; do not breast-feed if there are breast lesions; call healthcare provider for treatment; pump and dump breast milk till lesions are healed

Syphilis (spirochete)	Transmission to fetus can occur at any stage of maternal disease; early, untreated syphilis results in spontaneous abortion, stillbirth, or perinatal death in 40% of pregnancies; primary/secondary syphilis results in 60%–100% transmission; early latent infection results in 40% transmission; late latent infection results in 8% transmission	Primary stage: painless, indurated ulcer(s) (chancre) of the skin/mucous membrane at infection site. Secondary stage: rash, fever, muco-cutaneous lesions, malaise, splenomegaly, headache, sore throat, arthralgia, and lymphadenopathy occurring 1-2 mo after primary stage. Latent stages (seroreactive, but without clinical manifestations): Early: latent infection acquired within the preceding year. Late: all other latent infections, after the first year. Tertiary stage: gumma formation and cardiovascular disease that may occur years to decades after the primary infection	Asymptomatic at birth or symptomatic at birth and within the first 4–8 wk of life; all organ systems involved: hepatitis; pneumonitis; bone marrow failure; myocarditis; meningitis; nephrotic syndrome; rash (palms, soles); bone lesions; rhinitis (snuffles)	Antibiotic: for neonates with central nervous system involvement, aqueous penicillin G 100,000–150,000 U/kg/d IV q 12 h for 7 d and q 8 h/d for a total of 10 d (lumbar puncture must be repeated every 6 mo till normal results); for infants without central nervous system involvement, penicillin G procaine 50,000 U/kg/d IM, in a single dose for 10–14 d; if more than 1 d of treatment is missed in either of the above regimens, the entire course of therapy must be restarted	Skin lesions and nasal secretions of congenital infection are highly infectious (until after 24 h of treatment); importance of contact precautions and hand hygiene (handwashing/hand rubs); importance of continued follow-up care at 1, 2, 4, 6, and 12 mo of age to evaluate growth, development, serum titers, complete blood cell counts, and cerebrospinal fluid examinations (if cerebrospinal fluid initially positive)

Abbreviations: IM, intramuscularly; IV, intravenously.

Data from Venkatesh M, Merenstein GB, Adams K, et al. Infection in the neonate. In: Merenstein GB, Gardner SL, editors. Handbook of neonatal intensive care, 6th edition. St. Louis (MO): Mosby; 2006, p. 569–93; and American Academy of Pediatrics. Influenza. In: Red book: 2006 Report of the Committee on Infectious Diseases, 27th edition. Elk Grove (IL): American Academy of Pediatrics; 2006.

Table 2
Acquired neonatal infections: viral, bacterial, fungal

Agent	Incidence	Perinatal Presentation	Neonatal Symptoms	Treatment	Parent Education
Virus					
HIV (the causative agent of AIDS)	Mother-to-newborn transmission rates: antepartal—treatment with antiretrovirals reduces transmission rate from 30% to 8%; intrapartal—70% is decreased with administration of antiretrovirals to mother/baby; postpartal —16% with breast-feeding. Increased perinatal transmission: high maternal viral load, low CD4+ lymphocyte count, advanced maternal illness, increased exposure of fetus to maternal blood, placental inflammation, preterm delivery, prolonged labor, and prolonged rupture of the membranes	At risk: IV drug users (MOC/FOC); promiscuity; gay/bisexual sex/multiple heterosexual partners; Haitian ethnicity; parental blood transfusion before 1985. MOC may be asymptomatic, so antenatal testing/counseling/treatment recommended[42,43]	Usually asymptomatic in the neonatal period	Antiretroviral therapy: zidovudine alone or in combination with other antiretrovirals started at 8–12 h of life and continued for 6 wk, PO, 2 mg/kg/dose q 6 h. Prophylaxis for pneumocystis carinii pneumonia (begun at 6 wk of life through 1 y of age or until HIV infection is excluded): trimethoprim PO 5 mg/kg/d and sulfamethoxazole PO 25 mg/kg/d in 2 divided doses for 3 consecutive days in a week. Early treatment (within the first 3 mo of life) of HIV-positive infants with antiretroviral drugs reduces mortality rate by 75%[43]	Live HIV virus present in human milk. HIV-positive mothers in developed countries are advised not to breast-feed because (1) formula is a safe alternative to breast-feeding, (2) water supply is safe, (3) breast-feeding doubles risk of postpartal transmission of HIV virus to the infant,[44] need for ongoing follow-up care and childhood immunizations; prevention of infections with hand hygiene, regular bathing/skin care, clean food preparation
Varicella	Congenital varicella syndrome (1%–2%) when mother has varicella at delivery and infection occurs before 20 weeks' gestation; nosocomially acquired infections by preterms born of susceptible mothers, infants severely preterm regardless of maternal status, and immunocompromised infants	Generalized, pruritic, vesicular skin rash with lesions in various stages of development and resolution (crusting), mild fever, malaise	Congenital varicella is rare: teratogen with malformations of limbs (atrophy); skin scars; central nervous system and eye abnormalities	Maternal infection within 5 d before or 2 d after birth may be fatal for the newborn; administer zoster immune globulin 2 mL IM within 72 h of birth	Importance of passive immunization with zoster immune globulin; teach parents to screen themselves and all visitors to the neonatal ICU, including siblings/others who have been exposed to chickenpox; they should not visit the neonatal ICU for 21-d varicella incubation period

Influenza A and B	For influenza A, several reported cases in neonates;[45–47] twin pregnancy a risk factor for neonatal influenza,[48] for influenza B prevalence unknown; two reported cases[49,50] both with staphylococcus epidermis sepsis before influenza B; in neonatal ICU, both A and B acquired from infected health care providers, parents or visitors; incubation period 1–4 d; maximum viral shedding in first 3 d, but duration may be as long as 7 d or much longer in young infants[50]	Pregnant women should receive the trivalent influenza vaccine in the autumn if they will be pregnant during influenza season;[51,52] immunizing pregnant women is the single most important factor in decreasing influenza and hospitalization of infants ≤1 y of age; maternal influenza immunization during pregnancy protects newborns from influenza by bestowing higher levels of specific immunoglobulin G antibodies; preterms may not have received sufficient amounts of these antibodies because of their shortened gestation[50,52]	Symptoms are indistinguishable from other causes of septicemia	Rapid diagnostic tests so that unnecessary antibiotics are not used and antivirals are administered[52]	Importance of infection control measures—do not enter the neonatal ICU if ill with any respiratory infection; use hand hygiene; droplets and contaminated fomites are infectious; influenza immunizations essential in neonatal ICU and for other health care providers, parents, and siblings of ≥6 mo[50,52]
Human papilloma virus (HPV)	75% of sexually active adults will develop human papilloma virus; most will have no symptoms and the immune system clears the virus before symptoms or detection; more than 30 types are sexually transmitted; human papilloma virus is one of the most common sexually transmitted diseases; neonatal human papilloma virus infection occurs after birth through an infected birth canal and has also occurred after cesarean section	Asymptomatic or presence of infectious genital warts; pregnancy is a cofactor in the malignant transformation of human papilloma virus–infected tissue	Human papilloma virus infection of the epithelium resulting in (1) laryngeal warts, (2) recurrent respiratory papillomatosis	Surgical removal (which may need to be repeated) is necessary	Gardasil is approved by the Food and Drug Administration as vaccine for the prevention of 4 high-risk strains of human papilloma virus: 6, 11, 16, and 18 (human papilloma virus 6 and 11 cause 90% of genital warts; human papilloma virus 16 and 18 cause about 70% of all cervical cancers; the 4 strains together cause a small percentage of vulvar/vaginal cancers). Gardasil does not treat human papilloma virus if already present; vaccination is recommended for routine administration to 11–12-year-old girls; also to girls as young as 9 y of age and women 13–26 y of age[53]

(continued on next page)

Table 2
(continued)

Agent	Incidence	Perinatal Presentation	Neonatal Symptoms	Treatment	Parent Education
Respiratory syncytial virus (RSV)	> 50% of infants with bronchopulmonary dysplasia/chronic lung disease are rehospitalized in the first 2 y of life, most often with viral respiratory infections. Risk factors: (1) preterms <32 weeks' gestation with bronchopulmonary dysplasia/chronic lung disease; (2) preterms with bronchopulmonary dysplasia/chronic lung disease <2 y of age requiring treatment within 6 mo of the start of respiratory syncytial virus season; (3) preterms 32–35-wk gestational age, are <6 mo of age, and who have ≥2 of the following risk factors: severe neuromuscular disease; school-aged siblings; childcare attendance; exposure to air pollutants, including second-hand tobacco smoke; (4) congenital abnormalities/functional disorders of the airway; (5) infants ≤24 mo of age with hemodynamically significant acyanotic/cyanotic coronary heart disease; (6) children with severe immunodeficiencies, either congenital or acquired; (7) history of respiratory syncytial virus infection.[54] Higher risk for respiratory syncytial virus bronchiolitis in infants with Down syndrome[55]	Mother/father/siblings or health care providers present with a "cold"	Pneumonia, bronchiolitis, and otitis media	Prophylaxis: palvizumab 15 mg/kg IM monthly during respiratory syncytial virus season (give first dose before onset of respiratory syncytial virus season); respiratory syncytial virus immune globulin (RSV-IGIV) 750 mg/kg intravenously over 3–4 h monthly during respiratory syncytial virus season. Total fluid volume of 15 mL/kg	Infection control principles to prevent respiratory syncytial virus: (1) good hand washing/hygiene, (2) restrict contacts with the infant (no one with a "cold") (3) avoid crowds—church nurseries, daycare, shopping areas, (4) reduce/eliminate daycare or use with <2 or 3 children, (5) eliminate second-hand smoke exposure, (6) stress importance of influenza immunizations for all high-risk infants (beginning at 6 mo of age)[50] and all infant contacts, (7) stress importance of monthly respiratory syncytial virus immunizations during respiratory syncytial virus season

Bacteria			
Chlamydia	Most common sexually transmitted disease; MOC may be asymptomatic or may have vaginitis, urethritis, cervicitis	Conjunctivitis at 1–2 wk after birth; pneumonia with staccato cough, tachypnea, hypoxemia, eosinophilia, otitis, bronchiolitis	Screen/treat pregnant women before birth through an infected birth canal; conjunctivitis risk: 25%–50%; pneumonia risk: 5%–20%	Conjunctivitis: erythromycin 50 mg/kg/d in 4 divided doses PO for 14 d. Pneumonia: azithromycin 20 mg/kg PO daily for 3 d; or erythromycin 50 mg/kg/d in 4 divided doses for 14 d	Screen/treat pregnant women before birth through an infected birth canal; teach parents the signs/symptoms of infantile hypertrophic pyloric stenosis, which has been associated with the use of oral erythromycin
Group B *Streptococcus* (GBS)	77.5% of GBS disease occurs in neonates <1 wk of age; 78.5% of these cases occur in the first 24 h of life;[56] 4% risk of infecting the neonate if risk factors for early-onset GBS are present:[57] (1) preterm/late-preterms (<37 wk) with obstetric complications, such as prolonged rupture of membranes ≥ 18 h, chorioamnionitis, maternal fever (≥ 100.4° F [38° C]), preterm labor, urinary tract infection, fetal distress, neonatal aspiration; (2) previous newborn with GBS; (3) African American ethnicity (4) young maternal age; (5) low antibody level to GBS capsular polysaccharide, indicating immunologic vulnerability Preterms are more at risk for developing GBS, but most (75%) GBS-infected infants are term infants; neonatal infection: 80%; early-onset mortality rate: 5%	MOC birth canal colonized (10%–30%); but MOC asymptomatic. Transmission: 1-in-100 chance of infecting baby if colonized at labor/ delivery	Majority (98%) of colonized newborns are asymptomatic; early onset (first 24 h–first week of life; 2% of colonized neonates) develop fulminate, multisystem illness (pneumonia; sepsis; meningitis),[58] signs and symptoms of neonatal sepsis; late onset (7 d–3 mo of life) present with sepsis or meningitis; acquired from mother at birth or from other infected carriers	CDC maternal intrapartum antibiotic prophylaxis: at least 1 dose of IV penicillin, given 4 h before delivery; incomplete adherence to maternal antibiotic prophylaxis may not prevent early-onset group B neonatal sepsis. CDC neonatal management guidelines:[56] (1) MOC with suspected chorioamnionitis: full diagnostic evaluation and empiric antibiotics pending culture results; (2) lumbar puncture (if feasible) if clinical signs of sepsis; (3) discharge after 24 h reasonable if ≥38 weeks' gestation, asymptomatic, ≥4 h intrapartum antibiotic prophylaxis, home observation adequate, all other discharge criteria met. Neonatal: observe for 48 hrs if MOC treated as above; if MOC not treated, do CBC, blood culture, and observe; for asymptomatic preterms, do CBC, blood culture, and observe; for symptomatic preterms, do CBC, blood culture, chest radiograph, lumbar puncture, and other related tests, treat/observe.	90% of early-onset neonatal GBS prevented by treating mother with IV antibiotics. Prevention: CDC guidelines for prevention of GBS infection:[56] (1) perform universal prenatal screening with vaginal/ rectal GBS cultures of all pregnant women at 35–37 weeks' gestation; (2) use risk-based intrapartum antibiotic prophylaxis strategy for women with unknown GBS culture status at the time of labor/ birth. Indications for intrapartum antibiotic prophylaxis: (1) previous infant with invasive GBS; (2) GBS bacteriuria during current pregnancy; (3) positive GBS screening culture during current pregnancy (unless planned cesarean section, absence of labor, or amniotic membrane rupture); (4) unknown GBS status and any of the following: (a) delivery at <37 weeks' gestation; (b) amniotic membrane rupture ≥ 18 h; (c) intrapartum temperature ≥38°C (≥ 100.4°F)

(continued on next page)

Table 2
(continued)

Agent	Incidence	Perinatal Presentation	Neonatal Symptoms	Treatment	Parent Education
				Empiric antibiotic therapy (for 48–72 h): ampicillin 50 mg/kg/dose IV q 12 h (sepsis), 100 mg/kg/dose IV q 12 h (meningitis); gentamicin 2.5 mg/kg/dose IV q 12–24 h depending on gestational age. If laboratory results/clinical presentation negative for sepsis, discontinue antibiotics. If symptomatic or laboratory results suggest sepsis, treat with antibiotics for 7–10 d; treat 14 d for meningitis	
Hepatitis B	High-risk mothers: Asian, African, Eskimo, Haitian, Pacific Islanders	History of maternal liver disease, IV drug use, exposure to blood in medical/dental settings; HBsAG mothers may pass the infection to their infants at birth	Asymptomatic; occasional acute fulminate hepatitis with elevated liver enzymes	Immunizations: Active: For newborns with HBsAG-positive and HBsAG-negative mothers, give 3 separate doses—as soon as possible after birth, at 1 mo, and at 6 mo, recombivax 0.25–0.5 mL IM, or energix-B 0.5 mL IM. Passive: For newborns whose mothers have acute type B infection or mothers who are antigen positive, give within 12 h of birth hepatitis B immune globulin 0.5 mL/kg IM	Immunization (both active and passive) is indicated for newborns whose mothers are HBsAG positive because most newborns at risk of becoming infected from their mothers are HBsAG negative at birth. Untreated infants become HBsAG positive 4–12 wk after birth. These infants become lifelong asymptomatic carriers or develop hepatitis B. Active immunization for newborns born to HBsAG-negative mothers is also recommended

	Incidence/Epidemiology	Maternal Signs	Neonatal Signs	Treatment/Prophylaxis	Nursing Considerations
Gonorrhea	Incidence of infection highest in females 15–18 y of age and concurrent infection with chlamydia may exist	80% of mothers are asymptomatic; symptoms include vaginitis, urethritis, endocervicitis	Purulent eye conjunctivitis at 2–5 d after birth; scalp abscess with use of internal fetal monitoring; vaginitis, disseminated disease with bacteremia, arthritis, or meningitis	Eye prophylaxis: Antibiotics: 1% tetracycline or 0.5% erythromycin ophthalmic ointment Silver nitrate: 1% solution Infants born to mothers with known gonococcal infection: for term newborns, give ceftriaxone 125 mg IV/IM × 1; for preterm/low birth weight neonates, give ceftriaxone 25–50 mg/kg to a maximum of 125 mg/kg	Eye prophylaxis prevents opthalmia neonatorum and blindness, is required by state law, and is administered after the first hour of life (to facilitate parent-infant bonding)
Tuberculosis (TB)	Resurgence of active disease in at-risk mothers: Asian, Native American, HIV positive; 4.4 cases per 100,000 people, the lowest tuberculosis rate on record in the United States	May be asymptomatic or have respiratory or systemic symptoms (fever, weight loss); mother with active disease should be separated from the newborn until not contagious (sputum negative with treatment)	Neonates whose mothers have only pulmonary tuberculosis are not infected as a fetus, but may be infected after birth by their mothers; congenital tuberculosis is rare but can occur after maternal bacillemia; signs and symptoms are those of neonatal sepsis and failure-to-thrive in infancy	Mother: isoniazid and rifampin with pyridoxine supplementation in pregnant and breast-feeding women. Newborn: isoniazid at 10 mg/kg/d. Active immunization: for selected infants at risk for contracting tuberculosis, give as soon as possible after birth bacille Calmette-Guérin (BCG) 0.1 mL intradermally and divided into 2 sites over the deltoid muscle	Teach parents infection control measures, including need for good hand washing and wearing of mask; infants require pyridoxine supplementation if they are treated with isoniazid or are breast-feeding from a mother being treated with isoniazid

(continued on next page)

Table 2
(continued)

Agent	Incidence	Perinatal Presentation	Neonatal Symptoms	Treatment	Parent Education
Methicillin-resistant *Staphylococcus aureus* (MRSA), including hospital-acquired (HA-MRSA) and community-acquired (CA-MRSA)	0.8% of population is colonized with MRSA (highest colonization in 6–11-y-old children and females >60 y of age;[59] 2%–5% colonization rate in nurses and other health care workers; 63% prevalence rate of MRSA; children of health care workers more likely to be colonized with MRSA,[58,60] MRSA increasingly prevalent in health care settings (63% in 2004);[58,60] from 2002–2004, there was an increase from 50%–83% in the incidence of MRSA infections. HA-MRSA associated with antepartal invasive procedures, postpartal mastitis, skin and wound infections; acquired in neonatal ICU from fomites, contaminated hands of health care providers, equipment, and breast milk. CA-MRSA is spread with parents, health care workers, siblings of those with no risk factors for HA-MRSA. Most often causes skin and soft tissue injuries	Mother may have mastitis; MRSA-positive breast milk with no symptoms, skin/wound infection, infection after antepartal invasive procedure; colonization increases risk of infection in both mothers and babies	Skin and soft tissue infections; abscess; bacteremia/septicemia/meningitis; purulent conjunctivitis; orbital cellulitis; necrotizing fasciitis; septic arthritis; subglottic stenosis[61]	HA-MRSA is resistant to more antibiotics; treat infections with vancomycin IV; add gentamicin or rifampicin for serious systemic infections[24] CA-MRSA infections are more susceptible to ciprofloxacin, clindamycin, gentamicin and trimethoprim-sulfamethoxazole DS (double strength), tetracycline, linezolid, and vancomycin with or without rifampin;[24] alternative drugs (such as trimethoprim-sulfamethoxazole, linezolid, quinapristin/dalfopristin, floroquinolones) should be used after susceptibility testing is complete and with consultation with a pediatric infectious disease specialist;[24] antibiotic therapy, in standard dosage regimens, should be administered for at least 10 d and may be necessary for ≥4 wk for serious or disseminated infections[24] Neither sulfa drugs nor tetracycline are used in the neonate or in the breast-feeding mother because of their effects on the neonate	Transmission by direct contact with parents, staff, infected skin lesions, contaminated fomites, overcrowding, poor staffing. Education to prevent/control spread of MRSA: infection control guidelines; contact isolation and universal precautions; strict adherence to hand hygiene guidelines;[62] cohorting patients, staff and equipment; screening all skin lesions; covering wounds with impermeable dressings; not sharing hospital equipment/supplies or personal care items

Fungus

Organism	Characteristics / Risk factors	Transmission	Prophylaxis / Treatment	Signs and symptoms	Comments
Candida sp (most common)	The second most common infection after 72 h of life for preterms <1500 g. Other risk factors: congenital anomalies requiring surgery; multiple/prolonged vascular catheterization; preterms <32-wk gestation age; antibiotic therapy; total parenteral nutrition >5 d; IL >7 d; LOS >7 d; use of histamine blockers; and endotracheal tube intubation.[63–65] 1% invasive fungal infection in VLBW infants[66]	None—nosocomial acquired infection in neonatal ICU	Prophylaxis:[67] Universal strategy: fluconazole therapy (3–6 mg/kg) for all VLBW infants. High-risk strategy:[68] fluconazole therapy for VLBW at increased risk for fungal sepsis (ie, colonization, prolonged broad-spectrum antibiotic use, cephalosporin use [third generation] total parenteral nutrition/IL, endotracheal tube, central venous catheter, previous septicemia, postnatal steroids) Antifungal therapy: amphotericin B 0.1–1 mg/kg/d IV, begin at lowest dose and increase daily as tolerated; amphotericin B lipid complex 1–5 mg/kg/dose IV over 2 h, begin at lowest dose and increase daily as tolerated; 5-flurocytosine (5-FC) 50–100 mg/kg/d PO every 6 h; fluconazole 12 mg/kg loading dose IV, then 6 mg/kg/dose over 30 min every 24–72 h depending on postnatal and gestational age	Signs and symptoms of neonatal sepsis; skin infections in VLBW infants may become invasive and should be treated	As more VLBW infants survive and use antibiotics, fungal septicemia in the neonatal ICU has increased and is associated with an increase in morbidity (neuro-developmental problems) and mortality. Antifungal prophylaxis in the VLBW reduces the risk of invasive fungal infection while raising the risk of fungal resistance. Prophylaxis strategy may be either universal or based on high-risk status

Abbreviations: CA-MRSA, community-acquired methicillin-resistant *Staphylococcus aureus*; CBC, complete blood cell count; CDC, Centers for Disease Control and Prevention; FOC, father of child; GBS, group B *Streptococcus*; HA-MRSA, hospital acquired methicillin-resistant *Staphylococcus aureus*; HBsAG, hepatitis B surface antigen; IM, intramuscularly; MOC, mother of child; MRSA, methicillin-resistant *Staphylococcus aureus*; VLBW, very low birth weight

Data from Venkatesh M, Merenstein GB, Adams K, et al. Infection in the neonate. In: Merenstein GB, Gardner SL, editors. Handbook of neonatal intensive care, 6th edition. St. Louis (MO): Mosby; 2006, p. 569–93; and American Academy of Pediatrics. Influenza. In: Red book: 2006 Report of the Committee on Infectious Diseases, 27th edition. Elk Grove (IL): American Academy of Pediatrics; 2006.

Complete Physical Examination (PE) by MD/ APN
Complete Blood Count (CBC) with differential and platelet count
Cultures of non-permissive sites (blood; CSF; urine; closed body cavity)
Chemistries: electrolytes, glucose, CSF (glucose/protein)
Arterial Blood Gases: acid/ base ; oxygenation
Gram stain

C-reactive Protein (CRP); serum procalcitonin level
Tests for presence of bacterial antigens/ endotoxins: CIE*;
LA**, limulus lysate
X-rays: chest; abdomen; joint

* Counterimmunoelectrophoresis ** Latex agglutination

Fig. 6. Components of a sepsis workup in the neonate. *Data from* Venkatesh M, Merenstein GB, Adams K, et al. Infection in the neonate. In: Merenstein GB, Gardner SL, editors. Handbook of neonatal intensive care, 6th edition. St. Louis (MO): Mosby; 2006.

or exclude without a lumbar puncture. The presence of meningitis also alters antibiotic therapy, follow-up care, morbidity, and mortality.[1,37]

TREATMENT

Antibiotic therapy is the cornerstone of treatment for both presumed and confirmed neonatal sepsis.[1] After completing the sepsis workup, broad-spectrum antibiotics for coverage against both gram-positive and -negative organisms are *immediately* started.[1] Overtreatment of newborns with antibiotics is common because no set of universal signs/symptoms or diagnostic tests has been found to be reliable for very early diagnosis of neonatal sepsis. For every newborn with a positive blood culture, as many as 20 newborns are treated with antibiotics.[38] Usually empiric antibiotics, such as ampicillin and an aminoglycoside, are the drugs of choice pending culture and sensitivity results.[1,24] A recent study found an increased risk of death (double the mortality) from the use of ampicillin and cefotaxime versus ampicillin and gentamicin as empiric therapy for neonatal sepsis.[39] After the causative agent or agents and antibiotic sensitivities are identified, the best and least-toxic antibiotic and antibiotic combinations are started and continued for the recommended therapeutic course.[1]

Numerous physiologic derangements occur in neonates with severe infections.[5] Newborns with presumed or confirmed sepsis should be admitted to level II-III neonatal ICUs for observation of vital signs. Continuous cardiorespiratory monitoring should be employed to watch for apnea/bradycardia. Hypoxemia, which frequently accompanies sepsis, is monitored by continuous pulse oximetry and treated by the administration of supplemental oxygen to maintain the pulse oximetry saturations at 92% to 94%. Because septic neonates may develop hypovolemic or septic shock, their blood pressure should be monitored and, if necessary, maintained with volume expanders, inotropes, or both. Temperature instability (hypothermia or hyperthermia) may accompany infection and requires monitoring and documentation, placement in an incubator or radiant warmer for warmth (and observation) and maintenance of neutral thermal environment. Although the sick, infected neonate needs fluids and nutrition, use of the oral route is not safe because of paralytic ileus and the increased risk of aspiration. Thus, the infant should be placed on *nil per os* (NPO) status to indicate that nothing be given by mouth. Fluids, calories, volume, and medications should be administered intravenously. Septic neonates are also at increased risk for hypoglycemia, which needs point-of-care screening, treatment with intravenous glucose, and rescreening for efficacy of treatment. Foreign bodies (eg, peripherally inserted central catheter, umbilical artery catheter, umbilical venous catheter, Broviac catheter) need to be removed and cultured; abscesses must be incised and drained for antibiotic therapy to be effective.

SUMMARY

Quite reasonably, parents of infected newborns worry and need communication, emotional support, and instruction from all health care providers.[2] Primary nurses collaborate with families as "partners in care" to include parents in decision making and in direct care of their sick infants. Infection control should never be an excuse to exclude parents from caring for their infected infant.[5] No research has shown that the incidence of infection increases with involvement of parents, siblings, and family members, so long as they are taught proper infection control measures (eg, isolation precautions, hand hygiene.[1])

Prompt recognition, diagnosis, and treatment of the infected neonate results in improved morbidity and mortality. Both professional and parental caregivers must be knowledgeable about recognizing a "sick" baby, advocating for the infant, and ensuring that the infant receives timely interventions.

REFERENCES

1. Venkatesh M, Merenstein GB, Adams K, et al. Infection in the neonate. In: Merenstein GB, Gardner SL, editors. Handbook of neonatal intensive care. 6th edition. St. Louis (MO): Mosby; 2006. p. 569–93.
2. Lawn JE, Cousens S, Zupan J. 4 million neonatal deaths: when? where? why? Lancet 2005;365: 891–900.
3. The Young Infants Clinical Signs Study Group. Clinical signs that predict severe illness in children under age 2 months: a multi-center study. Lancet 2008;371:135–42.
4. World Health Organization. World health report 2005: make every mother and child count. Geneva: World Health Organization; 2006.
5. Gardner SL. "How will I know if my newborn is sick?" Nurse Currents 2008;2(2):1–5.
6. Pessoa-Silva CL, Hugonnet S, Pfister R, et al. Reduction of health care associated infection risk in neonates by successful hand hygiene promotion. Pediatrics 2007;120:e382–90.
7. Gardner SL. Late-preterm ("near-term") newborns: a neonatal nursing challenge. Nurse Currents 2007;1(1):1–7.
8. Rubarth LB. Nursing patterns of knowing in assessment of newborn sepsis [doctoral dissertation], University of Arizona, 2005.
9. Rubarth LB. Infants in peril: assessing sepsis in newborns. American Nurse Today 2008;3(4):14–6.
10. Gatchalian SR, Quiamboa BP, Morelos AM, et al. Bacterial and viral etiology of serious infections in very young Filipino infants. Pediatr Infect Dis J 1999;18:S50–5.
11. Lehmann D, Michael A, Omena M, et al. Bacterial and viral etiology of severe infection in children less than three months old in the highlands of Papua New Guinea. Pediatr Infect Dis J 1999;18: S42–9.
12. Muhe L, Tilahun M, Lulseged S, et al. Etiology of pneumonia, sepsis and meningitis in infants younger than three months of age in Ethiopia. Pediatr Infect Dis J 1999;18:S56–61.
13. Mulholland EK, Ogunlesi OO, Adegbola RA, et al. The aetiology of serious infections in young Gambian infants. Pediatr Infect Dis J 1999;18:S35–41.
14. The WHO Young Infants Study Group. Clinical prediction of serious bacterial infections in young infants in developing countries. Pediatr Infect Dis J 1999;18:S23–31.
15. Tulloch J. Integrated approach to child health in developing countries. Lancet 1999;354:516–20.
16. Weber MW, Mulholland EK, Jaffar S, et al. Evaluation of an algorithm for the integrated management of childhood illness in an area with seasonal malaria in the Gambia. Bull World Health Organ 1997;75: 25–32.
17. World Health Organization. IMCI chart booklet. Available at: http://www.who.int/child-adolescent-health/publications/IMCI/chartbooklet.htm. Accessed October 2008.
18. Källman J, Ekholm L, Eriksson M, et al. Contribution of interleukin-6 in distinguishing between mild respiratory disease and neonatal sepsis in the newborn infant. Acta Paediatr 1999;88:880–4.
19. LaForgia N, Coppola B, Carbone R, et al. Rapid detection of neonatal sepsis using polymerase chain reaction. Acta Paediatr 1997;86:1097–8.
20. Schelonka RL, Chai MK, Yoder BA, et al. Volume of blood required to detect common neonatal pathogens. J Pediatr 1996;129:275–8.
21. Sanghvi KP, Tudehope DI. Neonatal bacterial sepsis in a neonatal intensive care unit: a 5 year analysis. J Paediatr Child Health 1996;32:333–8.
22. Johnson CE, Whitwell JK, Pethe K, et al. Term newborns who are at risk for sepsis: are lumbar punctures necessary? Pediatrics 1997;99:E10.
23. Manroe BL, Weinberg AG, Rosenfeld CR, et al. The neonatal blood count in health and disease. I. Reference values for neutrophilic cells. J Pediatr 1979;95: 89–98.
24. American Academy of Pediatrics. Influenza. In: Red book: 2006 Report of the Committee on Infectious Diseases. 27th edition. Elk Grove (IL): AAP; 2006.
25. Christensen RD, Rothstein G, Hill HR, et al. Fatal early onset group B streptococcal sepsis with normal leukocyte counts. Pediatr Infect Dis J 1985;4:242–5.
26. Engle WD, Rosenfeld CR. Neutropenia in high risk neonates. J Pediatr 1984;105:982–6.
27. Benitz WE, Han MY, Madan A, et al. Serial serum C-reactive protein levels in the diagnosis of neonatal infection. Pediatrics 1998;102:E41.
28. Chan DK, Ho LY. Usefulness of C-reactive protein in the diagnosis of neonatal sepsis. Singapore Med J 1997;38:252–5.
29. Da Silva O, Ohlsson A, Kenyon C. Accuracy of leukocyte indices and C-reactive protein for diagnosis of neonatal sepsis: a critical review. Pediatr Infect Dis J 1995;14:362–6.
30. Philip AG, Mills PC. Use of C-reactive protein in minimizing antibiotic exposure: experience with infants initially admitted to a well-baby nursery. Pediatrics 2000;106:E4.
31. Berner R, Niemeyer CM, Leititis JU, et al. Plasma levels and gene expression of granulocyte colony-stimulating factor, tumor necrosis factor-alpha, interleukin (IL)-1beta, IL-6, IL-8, and soluble intercellular adhesion molecule-1 in neonatal early onset sepsis. Pediatr Res 1998;44:469–77.
32. Creech C, Kernodle D, Alsentzer A, et al. Increasing rates of nasal carriage of methicillin-resistant Staphylococcus aureus in healthy children. Pediatr Infect Dis J 2005;24:617–21.

33. Jaye DL, Waites KB. Clinical applications of C-reactive protein in pediatrics. Pediatr Infect Dis J 1997; 16:735–46.

34. Philip AG, Hewitt JR. Early diagnosis of neonatal sepsis. Pediatrics 1980;65:1036–41.

35. Clyne B, Olshaker JS. The C-reactive protein. J Emerg Med 1999;17:1019–25.

36. Chiesa C, Pacifico L, Mancuso G, et al. Procalcitonin in pediatrics: overview and challenge. Infection 1998;26:236–41.

37. Remington JS, Klein JO. Infectious diseases of the newborn infant. 5th edition. Philadelphia: WB Saunders; 2001.

38. Griffin MP, Moorman JR. Toward the early diagnosis of neonatal sepsis and sepsis-like illness using novel heart rate analysis. Pediatrics 2001;107:97–104.

39. Clark RH, Bloom BT, Spitzer AR, et al. Empiric use of ampicillin and cefotaxime, compared to ampicillin and gentamicin, for neonates at risk for sepsis is associated with an increased risk of neonatal death. Pediatrics 2006;117:67–74.

40. McLeod R, Boyer K, Karrison T, et al. Outcome of treatment for congenital toxoplasmosis, 1984–2004: The National Collaborative Chicago-Based Congenital Toxoplasmosis Study. Clin Infect Dis 2006;42:1383–94.

41. Centers for Disease Control and Prevention. Cytomegalovirus (CMV) and pregnancy: facts and prevention. Available at: www.cdc.gov/ncbddd/pregnancy_gateway/infection_CMV.htm. Accessed October 2008.

42. American Academy of Pediatrics, Committee on Pediatric AIDS. Perinatal human immunodeficiency virus testing and prevention of transmission. Pediatrics 2000;106:e88.

43. Volari A. Presentation at International AIDS Society conference in August 2007—Early treatment of HIV-infected infants reduces mortality risk—results of the CHER study.

44. Read JS. Human milk, breastfeeding, and transmission of human immunodeficiency virus type 1 in the United States, American Academy of Pediatrics Committee on Pediatric AIDS. Pediatrics 2003;112:1196–205.

45. Meibalane R, Sedmack GV, Sasidharan P, et al. Outbreak of influenza in a neonatal intensive care unit. J Pediatr 1977;91(6):974–6.

46. Wilkinson YS, Buttery JP, Andersen CC. Influenza in the neonatal intensive care unit. J Perinatol 2006;26:772–6.

47. Cunney RJ, Bialachowski A, Thornley D, et al. An outbreak of influenza A in a neonatal intensive care unit. Infect Control Hosp Epidemiol 2000;21:449–54.

48. Yusuf K, Soraisham AS, Fonseca K. Fatal influenza B virus pneumonia in a preterm neonate: case report and review of the literature. J Perinatol 2007; 27(10):623–5.

49. van den Dugen FA, van Furth AM, Fetter WP, et al. Fatal case of influenza B virus pneumonia in a preterm neonate. Pediatr Infect Dis J 2001;20(1):82–4.

50. American Academy of Pediatrics, Committee on Infectious Diseases. Prevention of influenza: recommendations for influenza immunization of children, 2007-2008. Pediatrics 2008;121:e1016–31.

51. Healy CM, Baker CJ. Prospects for prevention of childhood infections by maternal immunizations. Curr Opin Infect Dis 2006;19:271–6.

52. Centers for Disease Control and Prevention (CDC). Prevention and control of influenza–recommendations of the Advisory Committee on Immunization practices (ACIP). MMWR 2008. Available at: www.cdc.gov/flu. Accessed October 2008.

53. Centers for Disease Control and Prevention (CDC). Quadrivalent human papillomavirus vaccine—recommendations of the Advisory Committee on Immunization Practices (ACIP). MMWR 2007. Available at: www.cdc.gov/std/HPV/STDFact-HPV-vaccine.htm. Accessed October 2008.

54. American Academy of Pediatrics, Committee on Infectious Diseases and Committee on Fetus and Newborn. Revised indications for the use of palivizumid and RSV-IGIV for the prevention of respiratory syncytial virus infections. Pediatrics 2003;112:1442–6.

55. Bloemers BL, van Furth AM, Weijerman ME, et al. Down syndrome: a novel risk factor for respiratory syncytial virus bronchiolitis—a prospective birth-cohort study. Pediatrics 2007;120:e1076–81.

56. Centers for Disease Control and Prevention (CDC). Prevention of perinatal group B Streptococcal disease. MMWR 2002;51(RR11):1. Available at: www.cdc.gov/mmwr/preview/mmwrhtml/rr5111a1.htm. Accessed October 2008.

57. Carbonell-Estrany X, Figueras-Aloy j, Salcedo-Abizanda S, et al. Probable early-onset group B streptococcal neonatal sepsis: a serious clinical condition related to intrauterine infection. Arch Dis Child Fetal Neonatal Ed 2008;93:F85–9.

58. Haley R. Methicillin-resistant Staphylococcus aureus: do we just have to live with it? Ann Intern Med 1991;114:162–4.

59. Centers for Disease Control and Prevention (CDC). Methicillin-resistant Staphylococcus aureus (MRSA). Available at: www.cdc.gov/ncidod/aip/research/mrsa.html. Accessed October 2008.

60. National Nosocomial Infections Surveillance (NNIS) system report, data summary from January 1992 through June 2003, issued August 2003. Am J Infect Control 2003;31:481–98.

61. Gardner SL. Methicillin-resistant Staphylococcus aureus (MRSA) infections in maternal-newborn nursing practice. Nurse Currents 2008;1(2):1–7.

62. Romero D, Treston J, O'Sullivan A. Hand-to-hand combat: preventing MRSA infection. Nurse Pract 2006;31:16–8, 21–3.

63. Feja KN, Wu F, Roberts K, et al. Risk factors for candidemia in critically ill infants: a matched case-control study. J Pediatr 2005;147:156–61.

64. Manzoni P, Farina D, Leonessa M, et al. Risk factors for progression to invasive fungal infections in preterm neonates with fungal colonization. Pediatrics 2006;118:2359–64.

65. Saiman L, Ludington E, Dawson JD, et al. Risk factors for Candida species colonization of neonatal intensive care unit patients. Pediatr Infect Dis J 2001;20:1119–24.

66. Clerihew L, Lamagni TL, Brocklehurst P, et al. Invasive fungal infection in very low birthweight infants: national prospective surveillance study. Arch Dis Child Fetal Neonatal Ed 2006;91:F188–92.

67. Clerihew L, Austin N, McGuire W. Systemic antifungal prophylaxis for very low birth weight infants: systematic review. Arch Dis Child Fetal Neonatal Ed 2007;93:F198–200.

68. McCrossan BA, McHenry E, O'Neill F, et al. Selective fluconazole prophylaxis in high-risk babies to reduce invasive fungal infection. Arch Dis Child Fetal Neonatal Ed 2007;92:F454–8.

Index

Note: Page numbers of article titles are in **boldface** type.

Crit Care Nurs Clin N Am 21 (2009) 143–148
doi:10.1016/S0899-5885(09)00017-3
0899-5885/09/$ – see front matter © 2009 Elsevier Inc. All rights reserved.

ccnursing.theclinics.com